2016

Author. Jay Kay

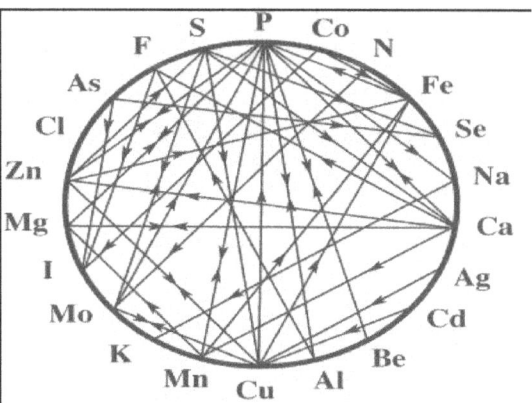

Fig. 1. Schematic illustrating how excesses of various elements can cause depression of other minerals.

Wake up to balancing your Nutrition

This book discusses various aspects of nutritional balancing program by combining ancient and contemporary techniques of rejuvenation based on revelations of Dr. Vethathiri and Dr. Wilson's approach. Let diseases become extinct in the history of mankind by liaising with Nature. Life is a quest for liaising with the eternal consciousness!

© Jay Kay 2016.

Published by
Jay Kay
writerjaykay@gmail.com

To my Gurus, Maharishi Vethathiri & the Buddha, Dr. Wilson for his insights. Many thanks to Mr. Muruganand, IT Project Manager, WellPoint, Los Angeles, USA who inspired me to write this book based on his real time life experiences of the nutritional balancing program.

Finally, my family, friends & publishers with gratitute... and above all my Divine Nature throbbing in me!

Thank you for all your patience and guidance...

Nutritional Balancing!

Dharma, speaks truth,
Its Organic is your Nature!
Pledge thy not,
Harm anyone by words, actions & deeds!

Oh my body-mind and spirit is Nature,
In five elements,
That summons itself;

Wonder, as my voice and the inner system
speaketh truth,
In my anonymous sleep can help!

For all mind things
It reacts like a precise machine!
With cause somewhere,
I am the reaction;

Inherent manifestations of the Divine,
As human consciousness,
With five elements maketh truth;
Body-mind & spirit;
Thou, heal thy self!

-   Jay kay

PREFACE

The ultimate human physiology has evolved over a million years from a single sense to the six senses. Nature has manifested as consciousness in human beings with every cell carrying the intelligence of the designer. It's like an artist immersed in his own art. Thus, Nature has designed a delicate system with exemplary ease over a period of time. Our human body is a sophisticated mechanism with each cell functioning as a laboratory. It is an absolute symphony, until you mess with it. Yes, truth is that human greed for money has polluted core elements of Nature, viz.,

1. Land,
2. Water
3. Fire &
4. Air

Luckily, the fifth element akash aka energy particles cannot be polluted as it is not perceived by the mundane human mind. The fifth element is not just an atom, it is the basic element known as energy particles. These associations of energy particles form atoms, molecules and compounds.

I had an opportunity to discuss holistic approach with my brother-in-law, Mr. Muruganand Moorthy, an IT Project Manager works with Well point and lives in Los Angeles, USA. We discussed various topics from ancient yoga to the modern medicines with its pro's and con's. I liked the nutritional balancing program for its unique ability to let body rejuvenate by itself without any medications. Indeed, I'd like to include another dimension of psychological detoxification method to it as physique comprises of 10% reasoning for toxic matter in body and psyche contributes to 90% of toxic accumulations in the body. In my view to keep your body, mind healthy, you should be able to address both tangible and intangible toxins accumulated in body and mind.

Whilst, the nutritional balancing program addresses the primary concerns of the body, mind is something which seems to have been left out. I would like to add what Dr. Wilson has missed out this critical factor in this unique nutritional balancing program. Indeed, karmic influences plays a vital role in the formation of diseases in the body, mind. It's both integrated, whilst Dr. has left out the diseases and its source in the mental plane. It's on the level of body, which is essential but it is just a starting point.

I'd like to invoke blessings of my beloved spiritual Guru, Dr. Maharishi Vethathiri and the Buddha. All Siddhas of South India to bless each of you and heal your body, mind. One part Dr. Wilson addressed was primarily body as west is primarily outward bound, however Siddhas of the ancient India have analyzed body, mind and soul with its lineage to the cosmos, which you may call as Nature or God. Dr. Wilson seems to have skewed thoughts regarding the benefits of Vegetarian diet as he believes it as high on copper; however it is insane as Siddha's of India have proved living longer and healthier using prana energy which is another source of energy to the body. They had proved to live for over 1000 years, for example. Saint Bogar lived for over 1000 years, known as Yugas and Patanjali sidda.

I would like to invoke blessings of all great souls to guide me to share the visions and solution for all impending problems of the World. Indeed, each of the factors contributes to the global warming. All these benefits described in nutritional balancing can be achieved through practices of Yoga, meditation and following a proper dietary pattern. Point is that nutritional balancing program creates awareness and helps you to take it to the mental plan.

In my view, you should take the best practices of the nutritional balancing program and combine it with practices of Simplified Kundalini Yoga, founded by Dr. Vethathiri and Vipassana (The Buddha). It is unique as these ancient practices will heal you completely, however due to inorganic toxic wastes, it is essential to take necessary care of best practices such as nutritional balancing program. This is just the beginning, eventually if it leads to the path of liberation, then it will be the best approach. For example, you may start with the simple nutritional program and then elevate your body; mind and soul towards spiritual growth by completely align with Nature. The ultimate alignment with nature in every moment is called enlightenment.

These methods would help you heal body, mind holistically. However, in my view nutritional balancing is primarily focusing on the body with less emphasis to mind with spiritual progression, whereas in any yoga programs, it is the other way around with focus on body-mind as a holistic unit. It is not new for the Indian culture, as the entire culture has evolved based on living in unison with Nature. In this context, most of the facts that Dr. Wilson is trying to portray in this program is synonymous to the Asian-Indian culture. For example, eating food was a meditation. These are simple ways of living as part of the Indian culture such as eating satvic food (vegetarian) without harming any living being etc.

Also, Indian civilization is one of the oldest in the world that started from Indus valley. A lot of native Indians are not even aware of their cultural heritage. Dr. Wilson seems to have studied bits and pieces of yoga, meditation and used it as part of the nutritional balancing program. It doesn't sound as comprehensive enough, however it is a good starting point to keep body healthy. All these yoga, pranayama, panchakarma practices of Indian ways of living are basically to evolve spiritually and one cannot evolve to the fullest consciousness without knowing methods of keeping body healthy. I believe somewhere the cultural heritage is lost due to the invasions of Mughals and colonies of the West leading to lost culture.

Anyhow, due to Dr. Vethathiri' s ardent efforts, we have discovered most of it and it is suitable for anyone in the world. His unique practices would heal body, mind and spirit to evolve as eternal super-consciousness. This is possible if a practitioner is able to adhere to these methods diligently. Dr. Vethathiri has gone a step ahead in proposing one governance with unification of borders at the UNO, however the frozen brains of the greedy politicians cannot accept anything that is good for the people of the World.

A true democracy would blossom only if the people of the World are empowered. I insist, you should rise to the occasion against all odds of food adulteration, environmental pollution, chemical usage in agriculture and physical abuse using allopathic etc. A holistic view is required to protect nature and self. I am sure a rebel will take place by the people of the world to protect nature and self. The organic master, G.Nammalvar had transformed nearly 100,000 acres of land from urea based to Organic farming by creating awareness of ecological farming similar to that of permaculture. The revolution has started by the Nature to protect her and the human beings. These greedy politicians will come to an end as people of the World have realized the politics. Our children are intelligent enough to understand contaminated food, water, land and air and money isn't primary today as the world is walking with cancer.

Your body should be healthy to delve deeper into mind analysis and without mind analysis, any technique will remain inadequate. The end goal of human consciousness is to achieve fulfillment by liaison with the eternal consciousness. In my view a lot of hypothesis by Dr. Wilson sounds good, however how much of it is pragmatic is the question to ask. Perhaps, you can do a hair mineral test to analyze where you stand in terms of toxic chemicals and try combined techniques of yoga, meditation without harming yourself to eliminate this toxicity in the body. I am glad that Dr. was able to create awareness in the world as consumer we have limited choices. The entire world has to think alike as the human needs are one and the same, hence a certain level of awareness is required across the leadership in the world to propagate holistic ways of living, diagnosis, and food to save the planet and the human beings before it becomes extinct. If you keep polluting the planet, you'd eventually leave nothing for the next generations to come. These factors have been part of ancient ways of living in unison with Nature. However, lost due to rapid urbanization in the name of science and technology.

I would like to request every citizen of the World to realize the looming threats to Nature due to greedy politicians those who have commercialized and poisoned food. I would like you to insist 'FDA' in the United States to pass food bills to protect the World citizens. I request citizens of the world to eat nutritious food, balance body, mind with techniques of yoga and meditation to lead a life span of over 100 years.

Thanks to Dr. Wilson for creating awareness about the Nutritional Balancing around the World, though in principle, I do not agree to Dr. Wilson's hypothesis of Vegetarian diet high on Copper, home-opathy and many other factors, but I feel it is a good starting point to eat right nutritious food.

The objectives of this book are to help you understand the nutritional balancing program as a holistic approach to heal body, mind and enhance soul to promote yourself to an absolute well-being. Though, the objectives is to realize the poisoning due to Industrialization, inorganic food and environmental pollution, it is imperative to take action to eliminate toxic waste accumulated in your body.

I'd like to provide my candid feedback of this program based on my understanding to help you assess yourself and embrace the right methods. As you know, prevention is better than cure. At least you can form social forms to create awareness campaigns in respective part of the world. Eventually, Nature will help you in the campaign to alleviate from the sufferings.

Chapter 1

Introduction

T oday (Nov' 2016) as we speak, World has many problems with looming threats of food poisoining due to extensive chemical usage in agriculture and food adulteration, nuclear war and environmental pollution not even sparing crawling creatures on-land to the smallest jelly fish in the Ocean. How many of you are really aware of food that you had consumed for dinner last night that may have contained toxic metals in it. Are you shocked to hear that? Besides inorganic food, now we will need to deal with the toxicity in food due to environment pollution in land, air and water. Your food contains several toxic compounds, thus resulting in adulterated food. Over and above, you've added toxic compounds to polished rice, wheat, pulses and sugar to look good and the fabulous restaurants further decorate your inorganic chicken with toxic colors to look and feel better. Astonished?

Hair test mineral analysis known as 'HTMA' is a non-invasive trichology test that can help you analyze toxicity in tissues. By analyzing the imbalances in the body, a certified nutritionist will provide supplemental therapies to balance nutrition. These tests are conducted in USA and in India, Richfeel does trichology tests in major cities, India.

On the contrary, if you visit an allopathy doctor to heal you, instead he would give you additional shots to infect your body further. Unfortunately, fact is that allopathy can be used for treating cuts or wounds and not diabetes, asthma etc. These are not diseases. Allopathy treatment is an absolute abuse of nature and the body. They do not have any cure for cancer. Nature has meticulously designed your body, mind and soul with the capacity to extend beyond the boundaries into eternity.

As we are talking about Global warming, in-organic food with looming threat of another nuclear war around the corner and environment pollution. Do not be paranoid, there is something called 'hope'. I wish and pray for the welfare of the mankind. Our nations should transform as one nation for one world to survive against the greedy politicians and barbaric religious leaders those who divided people in the name of caste, color, creed and religion. All Nations should formalize common healing methods as it cannot vary from one country to the other.

Trust me; none of these issues such as pollution, poverty, greed for money exists in Nature. Nature ever loves. A simple phenomenon of a germinating seed in proper soil, water is a witness to this loving phenomenon of Nature. All miseries are all manmade. It is your conditioning at the roots of mind. Each of you're made of the same mass, hence the basic necessities are common for everyone. Nature is an absolute socialist, where its utilities are common for anyone in this planet. There is no need for any religion beliefs as it is a simple truth. God is the ultimate source; in science we call it as 'Unified Force'.

How can God be different for every religion? Also, five core elements known as pancha boothas are common for everyone. So let's stop all wars in the name of religion, country etc. Secondly, our basic human needs and rights are one and the same, then why do you need borders. It is possible to have a common healthcare, one governance, judiciary and political framework etc. It can be one and the same! All five elements are common regardless of where you live and what you do. Nature is a democrat. None can claim authority of land, air, water, fire and energy particles as none of these five elements are man-made. These are common entities and each of you can enjoy equal rights from America to Africa. It's ridiculous to claim a piece of land as country. Man should stop abusing Nature. It is possible to promote alternate source of fuel, energy and it is necessary for the mankind to slowdown to regulate metabolism.

The Asia-India has always promoted a culture of living in unison with Nature. For centuries people lived by worshipping Nature. There was no ambition to challenge Nature. Instead, the objectives were to live in unison with nature, without abusing it. As the human populace grew smarter in science and technology, we believe in challenging nature. Human endeavor has become more and more greed for money from burning fossil fuels, deforestation without realizing the perils of human extinction.

The entire fauna and flora are ruthlessly killed leading to a major ecological disaster. World should have one constitutional framework to protect nature. Anyone who cuts trees must be imprisoned. There is no mindful approach in developing countries, whilst developed countries have stopped nuclear energy and still exporting nuclear material to countries like India. This is insane as what you do in the backyard will come back to you as tornado at your reception. This is a simple law of nature. You cannot protect boundaries, instead the entire planet should be one boundaries as all borders are manmade, which is just insane. Also, it is important to stop religious outrage by declaring science of the Unified force to help every citizen of the world to realize the God force as one and the same. The constitution should amend changes to the framework to protect welfare of the people, all living beings around and the ecology. Any industry that harms nature should be banned. All produce anywhere in the world must be organic and all types of chemical fertilizers must be stopped effective immediately considering the number of cancer patients across the world.

You must stop any factory that kills animals for food and it should be against declared as against law. You must step in to protect one world, one nation with one religion, one judiciary, commerce and one culture. Our human needs are one and the same. It cannot be different for different human. One governance should take up responsibilities of agriculture, maintaining forests by avoiding one person accumulating too much wealth beyond his need. It should be a socialistic society for the people and by the people of the world. The science and technology should help individuals to harness nature to its fullest without harming her. Let the transformation begin in each of you!

With the advent of mobile phones, sparrows have become extinct. With more and more toxic chemicals in agriculture, your food has been adulterated. But it seems enticing to you seeking packed tuna which is mouth-watering, however you didn't realize the toxicity and metal in it.

You've consumed so many packaged foods, carbonated drinks, alcohol, smoking etc. with toxicity and the adulterated milk to say the least. It's getting worse than ever. You've abused body, mind without realizing truth. The entire Western culture will need a transformation from education to food system needs an overhaul; they should research ancient ways of Asian-Indian ways of living, education. For example, Indians seems to have understood values of using herbs, honey, turmeric, spinach, garlic, pepper, ginger, cumin, hing (asafetida)…East or West is just a geographical boundary in mind. All discoveries, inventions are common to the people of the world. These are the citizens who should enjoy good health, long life free from diseases by leading a life in unison with Nature.

These Westerners should slow down, learn cooking vegetables, porridge using ragi, dhal, pulses etc. It is a good source of protein, minerals etc. Teach these cultural values to the entire man-kind. The Indian food was served in a plantain leaf with seven tastes with necessary proteins, minerals and vitamins. Rice, wheat, Ragi are all good food with a lot of carbohydrates. Cow Ghee consists of elements to control bad cholesterol causing heart diseases.

Neither your allopathic doctors, nor pharma companies would advise a proper nutrition as they need more business to survive. I am not undermining great allopath doctors, those who're serving the society with a real intent, I am against a few those who're greedy and treat people for money. Some of these allopathic doctors have been promoting cancer, heart diseases, diabetes, arthritis, ADHD etc. Simple reason is to increase drug sales. Remember, none of the above is a disease. You can take a conscious choice by eating right food to get away from the so called allopathic doctors. You must stay away from these "bad" guys, those who have commoditized body, mind for their own benefits. As an exception, there are "good" guys promoting health. Let's appreciate these good doctors. As an immediate need, you must take conscious decision to eat right for yourself and protect your family. Let's wellness be your birthright and protest silently against respective governments to STOP using soda, fluoride water, hybrid seeds, biotech modified seeds and food adulteration.

These are simple revelations of truth that you'd realize, if you're able to meditate. It makes no difference to Nature, as each of you're so precious and unique by its design. You've been so delicately designed by nature to realize its origin and not to suffer due to diseases in the body. One might be an artist, whilst the other one might be a carpenter. It really doesn't matter to Nature. What matters is how much you harness the potential of Nature within you by living in unison with Nature. There are certain laws that you cannot violate. If you do, then you should be prepared to accept the outcome as results. Nature is not intentional in giving you pains, it's your lack of understanding the laws of nature, which works perfectly well. If you clap your hands, you'd hear sound as a result of transformation of pressure.

This is a simple phenomenon and it applies in everything. In most of the miseries in human life is due to excessive inordinate desires. Thus, The Buddha said drop all desires, and Dr. Vethathiri proclaimed dropping inordinate desires can help you lead a happy, healthy and long life. The human life is around ~120 years, if you're aligned with Nature. These Siddhas of India have extended by transmutation of sexual vital fluid, which holds countless billions of sub-atomic life-force particles. If it is intact, then the longevity of life can be expanded. Further, a siddha named saint. Vallalar has transformed his body into light waves using a specific transmutation of cells. These techniques existed in ancient India and the science of healthy and long life was possible in ancient India. Most of these scriptures still exist in bits and pieces. Vallar has proclaimed a satvic food without harming anyone, otherwise if your body is developed by consuming animal flesh, then inadvertently, you'd suffer from ailments as indicated in his poems.

The indigenous ways of healing in India was based on aligning with Nature. India had known only organic ways of living in unison with Nature. This is her intrinsic cultural heritage, however due to rapid invasions and colonization; it has lost some of her heritage and techniques used in ancient days. However, luckily some of these methods still exists as I have witnessed in literature and methods practiced across various parts of India.

There is an absolute need to safeguard each of you to remain healthy by learning contemporary ways of living. I don't mean techology can help you survive longer, instead learning the ways to leverage technology to harness the power of Nature without disburbing its rhythm. Sounds interesting?

All biotechnology, health care centers, allopathy and industrialization seems to be the culprit in spoiling nature with reduced healthy life span of human beings. Next time, when you teach your kids to study, instead ask them observe Nature around and respect her. With more and more species becoming extinct, if it continues, humans will also become extince in a century. You should ask children to harness Nature, without disburbing its rhythm. Teach them Yoga to live in unison with Nature. The science and technology is one dimension, there are other aspects that can only be perceived such as meta physics, life-force etc. Hence, analytical research is okay, but need another dimension to life, physiology and psychology. Without this connotation, life will ever remain unfulfilled.

Atleast, I believe in the next generation, who will think about eco-friendly products to preserve Nature in order to harnessing its full potential for a healthy life. I am sure saviors will arrive, scientists will arrive to help you understand the potential Nature and ability to lead harmonious life in synch with Nature.

You must identify alternate source of fuel, enable bio-degradable products to avoid any further damages to ecology. As we speak, our beautiful planet is getting warmer day-by-day. Hence, we should leave the planet without spoiling it any further. This is in the outer, a similar story is happening within you, in the body.

Of course, there is a possibility to live longer and healthier despite polluted environment, food and rapid urbanization etc. While, we worry about social aspects of pollution, food adulteration and war around the corner, It is imperative to learn techniques to remain healthy, live longer to be able to survive against all odds by living in unison with Nature. Yes, I'd like to call this possibility as 'Nutritional Balancing' combined with ancient yoga systems, which is a holistic approach to heal your body-mind and soul.

Nutritional balancing is a sophisticated, integrated system for healing the body at a very deep level. It is about 45 years old, and it uses principles from both ancient and modern healing arts to drastically increase the vitality level of the body.

It employs modern theories such as the stress theory of disease, metabolic typing, cybernetics, holography, fractal mathematics, chaos theory, biological transmutation of the elements, and other physics and engineering concepts. These are combined with up-to-date Western medical physiology and biochemistry. It's good to analyze and combine with the best practices of alternate healing methods.

I asked these following three basic questions within myself and it would help you research it further:

1. What are the major classes of Nutrition?
2. What are toxins in body?
3. What are tissues?
4. How does the body eliminates wastes?

In my view, the cellular reaction to the chemical changes should be analyzed in detail, More so at the sub-atomic particle to analyze the impact in all three layers of the body. You might have heard about Reiki healing or SKY magnetic therapy, these are operating at the third layer which will need to be analyzed in detail. Unless magnetic therapy is combined with the cell biology and technology, you'd not be able to treat diseases.

Let's start with analysis of nutrition classes required for body to maintain good health. To answer in simple terms, nutrition are essential elements required for body. It helps in metabolism, which is rate of conversion of food into energy. Toxins are metals that harm body. These tissues are group of cells that forms layers in the body such epithilium. I believe I have answered the above questions. Finally, body eliminates waste through excretory organs, skin etc. Hence, in my view, if you don't mess up with the body system, nature takes care of it.

However, with the Western style of fast food on the go, over ambitious thinking in winning business at the expense of others resulted in toxicity in the body, and over ambitious growth plans have ruthlessly resulted in de-forestration. It's all man-made, hence you got to be aware of what you eat.

As you know, body is made up of cells. Each of these cells is a laboratory itself. It performs a lot of activitites for absorbing minerals from blood stream to perform essential activities. A simple example is like a disciplined cop, every cell will perform its own functions. It absorbs required nutrients by burning necessary proteins in its kitchen called '*Mitochondria*' and remaining waste is collected as urea which is excreted via urinary stream. It's a symphony of action that happens in your body in every moment.

Now, you can imagine the no. of cops in your county performing their duties to safeguard your life. Billions of cells do perform its functions every day in and day out. It is amazing, isn't?

Each of these cells are whirling at a certain speed. If you further go deeper in analysis, cells are made of sub-atomic particles known as 'energy particles' known as vethon particles as mentioned by Dr. Vethathiri through his unique revelations of truth. Irony is that these sub-atomic particles cannot be identified by compound microscope as it is not visible and forms the basic unit of a cell. There is nothing static in physiology. I mean, these sub-atomic particles are whirling at a high velocity. Hence, it forms a centripetal and centrifugal forces. The centripetal force is attraction that keeps two sub-atomic particles tide to each other and the centrifugal force, which is the force that keeps it at a distance. Now, image the collection of these sub-atomic particles forming cells, which is turn forming organs and organs grouped in systems such as respiratory, digestive systems which is all constantly in a whirling motion and nothing seems to be static in the entire physiology and yet it is all held together by the static and dynamic forces.

I hope it is clear with the basic unit of sub-atomic particles to the organs. Furthermore, you'll need to understand bio-magnetic circuits formed. As stated every organ and its underlying cells, basic unit of sub-atomic particles are all in whirling motion. Hence, it forms bio-magnetic circuits. It's like a ripple wave formed by a particle, whirling in water. This phenomenon is applicable to your physiology as well. These bio-magnetic circuits are formed due to the whirling sub-atomic particles that forms whirling wave patterns in the entire physiology. This is what

Dr. Vethathiri named it as 'Yogon' particles or shadow wave particles in simple terms. You might ask a question, on which media are all these particles revolving. It's a great question...

These bio particles in the body are whirling in a media. Like a ripple wave in water as a media, your sub-atomic particles, which is the basic building unit is whirling on a media called 'Gravity' or 'Unified Force' as named by Dr. Vethathiri based on his revelations of truth. Further, Dr. Vethathiri had stated this static force as '**Unified Force**', which is also called as God particles. The same phenomenon of the unit called body, applies to the entire universe.

As stated by Dr. Vethathiri the entire Universe has orginated from the static force (Gravitational force) to the dynamic state. The sexual vital fluid holds these sub-atomic particles. The quantity and quality of th sexual vital fluid helps in longetivity. This is the key aspect of longetivity of life. Dr. Vethathiri has emphasized on the importance of moderation in food, rest, sex and work. Your thinking plays a vital role in biochemical reactions. You're constantly burning inside, thus laeding to several repressed emotions. These emotions play a vital role in diseases in the body and mental disturbances. If you do it in excess, it will lead to several disorders, needless to say the toxicity in various other forms.

This is exactly what has been transcribed in every literature in Asia-India. Indians called life as 'Leela' since it is a time concept. I mean, with time t=1, static became dynamic, thus resulting in formation of sub-atomic particles, atoms, elements, compounds etc. The western world has stopped at the physiology, without realizing the fundamental unified force that binds everything together. Hence, there is a lack of understanding in everything and science cannot complete unless scientists comprhend unified force through revelations of truth in meditation.

Perhaps, West is not aware of this phenomenon, thus leading to lack of understanding in a holistic treatment of body, mind. The first soul of the planet, Dr. Vethathiri has made it explicity by identifying lineage of mind as the extension of God. He has found mind as wave. In other words, when mental frequency is reduced in its super dynamic state, it can be reduced from active functioning from beta, alpha, theta and finally delta state closer to the static force. This static force is the 'Unified Force' as (God as Religion named). The ultimate expansion of mind in its primordial state will yield its orgin from single sense to the six senses.

The above phenomenon of self realization is called enligtenment. It is possible for each of you with practices of yoga, meditation to keep body, mind healthy. It has accumulated so much of karmic influences, which are patterns of actions of the past sequence imprinted in DNA and brain cells. Eventually each of it would pop up as you grow older. You must sublimate these karmic past influences, once your conditioning is erased, you'll be able to liaise with the eternal consciousness. Now, with the above understanding, if you're able to analyze physiology and psychology, you'd have a different way to analyze wellness.

Watch your eating habits, before it becomes toxins.
Watch your thoughts before it becomes actions..

Your body will need energy to do work. Hence, it is imperative to eat right and not eat what you think is right. Just imagine the amount of chemicals in Pizza, packed Tuna sandwich, Burger and soda. Your children will need to be educated on actual meaning of civilization, which is ways of living in unison with Nature. Hence, India worships Nature in the form of Sun God known as Shurya, Moon God aka Chandra, Indra, Vayu aka Air, Agni aka Fire, Land aka Bhooma, Varun aka water and rivers, lakes etc were worshipped too with same reverence. Shakti indicates the dynamic state of consciousness, whilst Shiva is the static state. The manifestations of shakthi in to multiple forms is explained as Kali. This may sound primitive at the surface, if you analyze a little bit you'd understand the essence of it with basic revelations of truth. This is the ultimate secret of the vedic truth. God is one and the same known as Unified Force. It can be named as Allah, Christ, Krishna or anyone. It's all one and the same. It has manifested from static state of consciousness to human consciousness. It have evolved over thousands of years. Hence, in Nature every living being has equal rights for survival and human beings cannot claim it for any reason unless it is for survival. These species had evolved from amoeba to the six sense human beings and there is no disconnect in the evolution till date. Finally, human consciousness has evolved to realize his own self and lineage to the ultimate nature. This is the purpose of life, which is also known as 'Leela' in hindu scriptures. It denotes the ultimate purpose of life.

The objectives of the epics, literature in India were to inculcate a cultural transformation of respecting nature and living in unison by harnessing it and not by jeopardizing it. In India, there were idols of god tied to trees, so many linga idol is attached to the roots of trees for a simple reason to protect nature. The enlightened souls have realized these aspects and the crooked mindness of human beings to chop trees without realization. Now, in modern societies, you feel ashamed of touching a bare naked trees and you'd detest cow dung and try to garnish your body with inorganic perfumes from head to toes. What non-sense is this? Is this a real civilization and growth ? The real abhoriginals who are not a typical gentlemen or women in suit seem to have better knowledge of living in unison with Nature. I am not sure if you've evolved culturally. What is the use of technology used for atom bombs to kill people in masses? From time immemorial,

India had taught religiousness to the world from Buddha, Boddhi Dharma rhode his horse to reach China to spread real CHAN over a period of three years via forests, which became ZEN meditation. So many of these enlightened souls of sddhas to Dr. Vethathiri tirelessly had embarked shores of far off East to inculcate a real culture. The contemporary mystics Bhagwan Osho, Vivekananda, Yogananda Paramahamsa, Dr. Vethathiri, Sri Sri Ravi Shankar and Jaggi Vasudev. Many more have ventured into far West to teach about the ancient cultural evolution of India. By nature, world is democratic, any discoveries to aleviate pain should be universal.

Indeed, you must stop teaching children about the great history of Alexander, Hitler, mussolini the massacre(s) to the world of Buddha, Bodhi Dharma, Organic Master, Dr. Nammazhvar and Dr. Vethathiri. The west should learn best cultural ethos from the East and the East should learn the best technology from the West. A contemporary human will be balanced in east and the west, the inner and the outer. There has been no separation in any boundaries by nature, it was man made. Hence, let's forget these boundaries and expand ourselves towards universal brotherhood. Otherwise, Western gun culture will spread like virus in children, leading to disaster.

In the name of rapid urbanization, many countries have ruthlessly destroyed forests and the eco system. The entire bio-diversity is in jeopardy sparing no country. Hence, the ecological disasters are universal and democratic for each of you, regardless of where you live in this blue planet. Now, let's analyze the classes of nutrition with its benefits. You'll need carbs, protein, fat, vitamins, minerals, and water for maintaing good health. Dr. Vethathiri has mentioned about various types of meditation. Each of these meditations techniques will help you in resolving deficiencies at the sub-atomic level and it helps you at subtle levels. For example, 9 center meditation will help you in balancing energy levels. Thuriyatheeth meditation will help you in aleviating karmic influences of the past. The unique ways of pancha bootha navagruha meditation (9 planet & 5 elements meditation) which is very powerful by allowing you to liaise with the planets. This is very unique to help you align with nature and manage nutrient deficiencies, especially in terms of mineral imbalance. Also, I thought about animals that does not go through any nutrient defeciencies. I have not heard of any monkey getting wilder due to Al or Cu! This needs extensive research on animals too in my view to realize the values of nutrient balancing. Since, animals are aligned with nature, perhaps there is no impact to the extent in human beings.

As Dr. Vethathiri has said, these meditative techniques work at the deeper root levels in the sub-conscious mind and it helps in streamlining core elements (water, air, heat & bio-magnetic circuit) in the right proportion. Indeed, this strategy of analyzing core elements is the fundamental aspect of maintaining good health. Any fluctuations due to excessive use of thoughts, actions would result in imbalance in the above core elements.

The modern medicines are focussed on harmones and nutrition without analyzing the fundamental aspects of the core elements highlighted above. These parameters play a vital role in chemical synthesis, which would eventually cause harmonal imbalance. For example, an excessive usage of thoughts as mental wave would result in wastage of bio-magnetic energy. This is turn would result in dissipating bio-magnetic distortion in the flow, thus resulting in short-circuits. Eventually, more and more energy would be wasted through this short circuits, causing long term illness. You'll need to stop this first and work at sub-atom level to treat diseases.

Once again to reiterate, Dr. Vethathiri's approach is at the sub-atomic layer to ensure all three layers of body are in sync. First step is to increase energy levels in this practice to boost immunity against diseases. Hence, Siddhic way of treating diseases was primarily at the sub-atomic levels which in turn helped in governance of minerals, fat and all other classes of nutrition. Once body is streamlined at the sub-atomic level, next point was to maintain good health by managing core elements in proportion. I believe these practices helped in maintaining good classes of nutrion in the body without actually having to eliminate toxicity in the body. This was unique to siddhic practices. There were techniques as discussed in the earlier section such as pancha karma to eliminate toxicity thorugh oil enema and light vegetarian food.

Classes of Nutrition

You know body needs energy and carbs provide a good source of energy. These are grouped into simple and complex. Well, simple carbs are sugars whereas complex carbs consist of starch and fiber. Well, what is it used for? It is primarily used for fuelling muscles and brain. The soluble fiber (fruits, legumes, nuts, seeds, and brown rice, and oat, barley and rice brans) lowers blood cholesterol and helps to control blood sugar levels while providing very little energy. The insoluble fiber (wheat and corn bran, whole-grain breads and cereals, vegetables, fruit skins, nuts) doesn't provide any calories. It helps to alleviate digestive disorders like constipation or diverticulitis and may help prevent colon cancer. Most calories (55-60%) should come from carbohydrates. Sources of carbohydrates include grain products such as breads, cereals, pasta, and rice as well as fruits and vegetables.

Next is protein from food is broken down into amino acids by the digestive system. These amino acids are then used for building and repairing muscles, red blood cells, hair and other tissues, and for making hormones. Your body needs immune to fight against diseases, hence adequate protein intake is also important for a healthy immune system. Because protein is a source of calories (4 kcal per gram), it will be used for energy if not enough carbohydrate is available due to skipped meals, heavy exercise, etc. Main sources of protein are milk, cheese and eggs and vegetable sources like legumes (beans, lentils, dried peas, nuts) and seeds. I do not advocate animal fat due to the damages done to the body at the sub-atomic layer and it will harm the bio-magnetic layer.

Fat plays an important role in a healthy diet. Fat maintains skin and hair, cushions vital organs, provides insulation, and is necessary for the production and absorption of certain vitamins and hormones.

Vitamins help to regulate chemical reactions in the body. There are 13 vitamins, including vitamins A, B complex, C, D, E, and K. Because most vitamins cannot be made in the body, we must obtain them through the diet. Many people say that they feel more energetic after consuming vitamins, but vitamins are not a source of energy (calories). Vitamins are best consumed through a varied diet rather than as a supplement because there is little chance of taking too high a dose.

These Minerals are components of foods that are involved in many body functions. For example, calcium and magnesium are important for bone structure, and iron is needed for our red blood cells to transport oxygen. Like vitamins, minerals are not a source of energy and are best obtained through a varied diet rather than supplements. Minerals form the base for the nutrition balancing program, where your toxicity metal content is analyzed and balanced as part of the program.

Most of our body weight (60-70%) is made up of water. Water helps to control our body temperature, carries nutrients and waste products from our cells, and is needed for our cells to function.

Dr. Vethathiri, an enlightened master has mentioned that food is transformed in to body as the following:

1. Juice,
2. Blood,
3. Fat,
4. Bone Marrow,
5. Bones
6. Muscles &
7. Sexual Vital Fluid (semen)

Wholesome food such as millets, rice, and wheat are all good for health along with cooked vegetables. It should be easily digestible. It can be millet porridge for breakfast with light Idli/dosa (rick pancake) with sambar (dhal porridge) or rice, wheat bread and then good meal for lunch comprising of wheat roti, rice, vegetables, proteins available in plenty in dhal, cow ghee with a lot of carbs in rice/wheat, curd, butter milk, spinach, organic egg (rich in protein) and fruits. Drink water as you need and feel thirsty and eat only when you're hungry. It is essential to take seven different types of tastes in food (sweet, salt, sour, bitter etc.) for maintaining chemical balance in the body. The quantity and quality of sexual vital fluid determine good health. If it is diluted, it would result in disease prone body. Hence, in ancient siddhic practices of kaya kalpa, they tried techniques of solidifying sexual vital fluid to be able to hold the sub-atomic particles to live longer for more than a century. It actually worked for them; however in this era of technological advancements, this may seem impossible. Dr. Vethathiri has further simplified in his SKY practices with few practices of kaya kalpa to ensure leading a life of diseases free body to live healthy, longer. Often times that you'd have noticed in siddhic practices the emphasis is on the subtle layer of the body than the physical, though both are important. There is a lot more going on in the sub-atomic level such as thoughts, desires, emotions and six temperamental moods (greed, anger, miserliness, immoral sexual passion, vanity & vengeance).

Each of it would result in dissipating enormous amount of energy. For example, Dr. Vethathiri used to state that if you're able to remain with an equanimity mind, then it is possible to regain huge store of energy in the body, mind. You'd need a certain state of mind to achieve peace. It is possible to achieve by practicing yoga, meditation or witnessing as stated by the Buddha.

Food is medicine and should be taken like a meditation and not gulping something while talking to someone over the phone. It will burn your stomach and heart. If you want to lead a healthy life style, then it is imperative to follow basic principles in life. You must avoid Maida, fish, red-meat, masala, too much caffeine, soda, chocolates; avoid fluoride tooth paste, soaps and munching habits due to toxicity. It's insane for countries like India leaning on to Western lifestyle and it is a welcome change to see western countries changing its lifestyle in to yoga and vegetarian diet. As discussed in the previous section, even the sub-atomic particles are disturbed by the mental wavelength of the person, who is serving food. Hence, it is essential to maintain a calm mind while consuming food. It should be in a good sitting posture and relaxed without much talking and thinking as food is medicine. You must give its due attention without over eating or starving. You must eat food only when really hungry; perhaps you can take food after 45 minutes – 1 hour after you really feel hungry. This would prepare the physiology with necessary fluids in the body secreted prior to your meal. You must stop eating junk food, processed meat etc. These are very toxic and it will harm your body.

As a highlight of the program, Dr. Vethathiri has formulated techniques to eliminate toxins deeper in the sub-conscious mind through silence, thoughts analysis, moralization of desire and contemplation of 'Who Am I?' These are all crisp practices based on the siddhic tradition and heritage of India. Perhaps, Dr. Wilson can study these techniques to enhance the nutritional balancing program, which sounds like just the body based, whereas 90% of toxins are based on the accumulated karmic influences, which Dr. Wilson has no idea about these factors causing significant chemical reaction in the body, thus resulting in diseases. Apparently, changing food pattern is a good start, however it cannot lead you to a holistic plan to resolve all conflicts in body, mind.

Typically, Asian-Indian meal is considered to be a balanced food with good intake of carb, proteins, fat and minerals. Some of you would have witnessed your grand-parents, would have lived over 80+ years of life span on an average. This is due to good physical exercise, simple meditation and good diet as described. India was predominantly dependent on ecological Agriculture and this culture is being lost. The usage of urea is leading to an ecological disaster, with the plight of farmers in India in jeopardy. The western world taught these poor farmers about chemical fertilizers to increase yield/hectare.

The ecological farming and living in unison with nature are part of the Indian culture and nothing new, until west imposed its food habits changing the dietary habits, thus leading to sedentary life-style resulting in diseases in the body. Its' time to wake-up and train your children in ecological agriculture, farming, simplified yoga and meditation at an early stage. India has its cultural heritage to teach the entire world. I believe Dr. Wilson didn't find time to analyze ancient Asian Indian ways of living, where they had proved to extend life for centuries, yugas by solidification of sexual vital fluid, which is the source of life.

Perhaps, Dr. Wilson could have analyzed hair strand of an enlightened master from India, China, and Japan ZEN or anywhere in the world, which could have been a benchmark. Perhaps, trying hair mineral analysis of an enlightened soul will yield a different story.

Dr. Vethathiri has indicated if you're deficient in any of the vitamins, minerals. Of course, you'll need nutritious food to keep body healthy. But the quantity is dependent on the quanta of work. If you eat rich food without enough work would result in obesity with a lot of stocked calories without burnt. Thus, a lot of residue is formed in the body, resulting in toxins. The best way is to fast once a while to rejuvenate your body. You might have observed dogs sometimes taking leaves to heal themselves if there is a digestive problem. It will not eat until its stomach is completely cured. Only humans lose awareness in every meal, to enjoy food for mundane pleasures alone. It's not bad, but must realize it in a state of awareness. Otherwise, you'd overeat over and over again, despite several experiences.

Through fasting, you'd allow body to absorb necessary nutrients. Further, Dr. Vethathiri's practices such as relaxation, acupressure, massage and kundalini meditation is a wholesome and holistic approach to heal body, mind and soul. Also, it will help you progress towards eternal consciousness.

The nine center meditation focusses on various chakras, which are the gland centers as well. For example, focusing between eye-bro's helps you in regulating pituitary gland. The crown chakra helps in regulating pineal gland. Also, nine center planetary meditations would help in liaising with respective planets like mercury, Saturn to resolve mineral deficiencies. You're so organically connected with Nature; hence you should perhaps allow nature to heal you at times. Thus, fasting can resume from many issues. Each of it helps you in maintaining hormone levels. The hormones secreted by pituitary gland helps in regulating blood pressure, thyroid gland, sex glands and conversion of food into energy (metabolism).

Hence, Dr. Vethathiri has advised several aspirants to practice meditation by focusing between eye-bro on the pituitary gland, which helps in regulating metabolism. Dr. Vethathiri's techniques involve keeping a healthy body, mind to enhance soul to eternity. Further, his pledge for one governance at UNO would help us consolidate borders, to stop spending in wars and utilize funds to eradicate poverty, diseases etc. A simple relaxation, acupressure techniques followed in Dr. Vethathiri SKY practices will help in streamlining bio-magnetic circuit. Further, heat, air and water circulation can be streamlined in few asana. For example, Makara Sana focuses on spinal cord and hand, leg exercises will help you in maintain proper blood circulation. Most of the diseases in the body are due to short circuit in the body are primarily due to lack of flow of blood, heat, air, water and bio-magnetic flow in the body.

Dr. Vethathiri has identified these deficiencies can be resolved by liaison with cosmic consciousness. Also, fasting is a good technique to allow nature to fill in mineral deficiencies. In a deeper state of meditation, the cosmic consciousness will heal the body. Also, pancha booth meditation will help in liaison with five elements and nine planets that would fill in required minerals in the body. I have my own doubts, if Dr. Wilson has ever analyzed these facts.

Also, there are ways in ancient India such as panchakarma to eliminate toxins in the body. According to Ayurveda, the unique therapy of Panchakarma (meaning five actions) completely removes toxins from the body and mind. This method reverses the disease path from its manifestation stage, back into the blood stream, and eventually into the gastro-intestinal tract. It is achieved through special diets, oil massage, and steam therapy. At the completion of these therapies, special forms of emesis, purgation, and enema remove accumulated doshas from their sites of origin. Finally, Ayurveda rejuvenates-rebuilding the body's cells and tissues after toxins are removed. I think Dr. Wilson has not studied this technique in detail. Now, let's understand this ancient Indian technique known as Panchakarma as described below.

Panchakarma Technique

It is basically a technique followed in ancient Asia-India to remove toxins in your body. You will have to consult a Dr. to discuss health concerns and goals. Dr. will prescribe herbs, stress relief techniques, a lifestyle routine and Ayurveda protocols to help remove the root cause of your symptoms and prepare you for Panchakarma.

There is a period of seven days preparation known as Oleation, which is cleanse process that you can do it at home. Oleation helps you enter fat metabolism mode, pulls toxins from deep within your tissues to your digestive system for removal, balances blood sugar (and thus mood and energy), improves digestion, and opens your detox channels. Each morning you will drink increasing amounts of melted ghee, then follow a nonfat diet of khichadi (rice and beans), with steamed veggies and lean protein as needed. Oleation is easy for most people to do while working and continuing their regular life, though it does require some commitment. On the last day of Oleation, you will do a gentle laxative to remove any toxins that have accumulated in the intestinal tract.

During Panchakarma

Panchakarma is an experience of transformation. You will experience a renewed sensation of healing from within, a powerful and potentially life-changing exchange of energy in your body, rejuvenating your spirit and soothing your soul. Each of the daily treatments you will be receiving, are designed to bring you into a deep experience of release. Each person will have different experiences. You may feel tired and experience a small amount of bloating or heaviness. As you progress, in next couple of days, you may possibly feel a little lethargic and fatigued. This will pass as the liver is working hard to filter the blood of toxins. Emotions may feel engaged more than usual. Old memories may surface. Use the time to journal and release any emotional toxins that you have accumulated. Remember, the mind and body accumulates toxic build-up. Take it very easy and drink plenty of hot water and/or ginger tea. Whatever is happening, know that the body is deeply cleansing all toxins from the body. Continue to eat lightly and get plenty of rest. The Rounding Program of yoga asana and pranayama will greatly enhance and smooth the process of purification. Finally, you'd start feeling lighter and lighter.

Basti (Oil Enema) During Panchakarma

During your Panchakarma you will receive instructions to give yourself a Basti, or herb-infused oil enema, each evening before bed. The Basti is designed to rejuvenate and nourish the colon tissue. The LifeSpa Basti is a warm oil and herbal decoction enema that gently nourishes and rejuvenates the tissues of the colon, which generally experience excess air and dryness. Each Basti is a unique experience, so listen to your body and go when you need to. There should not be any cramping, diarrhea or forced elimination. This should be gentle and easy for you. If you experience any discomfort please let us know.

General Guidelines during Panchakarma

It is advised to get plenty of rest and to avoid strenuous exercise, sexual activity, late nights, loud music, television and other such stimulating activities. The only exercise we advise is the gentle yoga stretches that Dr. will give to you on your first day. Running, hiking, biking are all too strenuous for this week when we are trying to get you to turn down the volume, and let your body detox. It is also advised to take particular care to keep warm and protect you from wind and excessive sunlight.

Observe your thoughts and experiences and follow the self-inquiry guidance Dr. suggests. Eat somewhat less quantity than usual (between ½ to ¾ of capacity) and continue to eat khichari. You can add steamed vegetables and a little bit of high quality fat during Panchakarma. In the next section, let's analyze excretory system in the body as illustrated below in Figure 1-1.

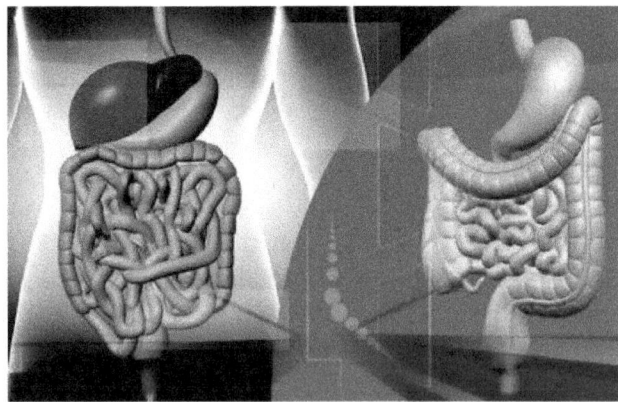

Figure 1-1 Excretory system (Intestines)

The above Figure 1-1 illustrates intestines.

The excretory system is a system of organs that removes waste products from the body. When cells in the body break down proteins (large molecules that are essential to the structure and functioning of all living cells), they produce wastes such as urea (a chemical compound of carbon, hydrogen, nitrogen, and oxygen). When cells break down carbohydrates (compounds consisting of carbon, hydrogen, and oxygen and used as a food), they produce water and carbon dioxide as waste products. If these useless waste products are allowed to accumulate in the body, they would become dangerous to the body's health. The kidneys, considered the main excretory organs in humans, eliminate water, urea, and other waste products from the body in the form of urine.

Other systems and organs in the body also play a part in excretion. The respiratory system eliminates water vapor and carbon dioxide through exhalation (the process of breathing out). The digestive system removes feces, the solid undigested wastes of digestion, by a process called defecation or elimination. The skin also acts as an organ of excretion by removing water and small amounts of urea and salts (as sweat).

Urinary system

The kidneys are bean-shaped organs located at the small of the back near the spinal column. The left kidney sits slightly higher than the right one. The size of an adult kidney is approximately 4 inches (10 centimeters) long and 2 inches (5 centimeters) wide. To maintain human life, it is necessary for at least one of the kidneys to function properly.

Blood carries waste products to the kidneys via the renal artery. Inside each kidney, blood is transported to 1.2 million filtering units called nephrons (pronounced NEFF-rons). The cells in nephrons take in the liquid portion of the blood and filter out impurities (urea, mineral salts, and other toxins). Necessary substances such as certain salts, water, glucose (sugar), and other nutrients are returned to the blood stream via the renal vein.

Development. Symptom removal and eradication of diseases of all kinds are wonderful, but one can go beyond this level of healing. Nutritional balancing is development science. Development is a unique process that is natural to human beings, but does not occur often because the bodies are malnourished, and drug medicine and most nutritional programs do not provide the nutrients and conditions needed for development.

Development increase one's mental functioning, improves the immune response far above that which most people achieve with any other healing program, and can extend life. This exciting topic is discussed in other articles on this website such as Development.

Nutritional balancing is not a remedy science, and does not involve the diagnosis of diseases. In this way, it differs markedly from modern allopathic medicine, as it doesn't suppress diseases with antibiotics. Remedies are simply not needed, in almost all cases, if one balances the body properly.

In nutritional balancing, diagnosis of diseases is not needed, either, in almost all cases. However, if one renourishes and balances the body chemistry properly, most diseases and symptoms simply vanish. This is in sync with ancient yoga practices, where they treated holistically and not the diseases. The human body was induced with external herbs to generate required antigens to fight these diseases. There was no side effects in these practices aligned with Nature as it helps your body produce its defence mechanism. Allopathy abrupts with the natural healing and its inherent defence mechanism. Dr.Vethathiri's SKY practice is based on the study of over 50+ years of an Enlightened soul based on his extensive expertise in homeopathy, ayurvedic treatment and studying ancient literature.

Dr. Vethathiri's approach is a holistic one with balancing body, mind and soul by leveraging practices of SKY exercies known as asanas, with postures every cell is re-aligned. Also, kaya kala exercises rejuvenates sexual vital fluid, which is like a battery to the whole body. This exercise will boost your energy levels if practiced consistently. It generates countless billions of sub-atomic particles. Finally, meditation and introspective analysis to heal

48

conditioning in mind and it works at sub-concscious layers to eliminate any toxins accumulated in the body. If you carefully assess these techniques of asanas, kriyas, it helps you to balance emotions, streamline blood, heat, air, magnetic circuits in the body. This will aleviate all problems. Thus, you'd be able to restore complete metabolism.

Dr. Vethathiri has prescribed a simple vegetarian meal such as millets, vegetables and wholesome wheat, rice to ensure a balanced diet. But the rule is to be aware while you eat food to ensure you'd never exceed the limits. The emphasis is to maintain limits in food, work, sex and rest. This is the secret for a healthy living. If you exceed, then you'd end-up in all sorts of disorders in the body, mind, thus leading to diseases in the body. You should practice regularly with a simple nutritious diet to keep body, mind healthy. Also, it is essential to take a week long silence practices to ensure it works at the deeper levels to eliminate karmic influences. These are karmas accumulated from the past generations stored as strands of magnetics strips in the body cells, mind and organs. It is possible to eliminate with consistent practices of introspection and meditation. If the cellular alignment is distorted, this will lead to several issues eventually.

Once again, Dr. Vethathiri was very particular about emotional well being. Each of these thoughts induced in brain cells will invoke a certain environment in the body, resulting in bio-chemical changes. It's the law of Nature. As a conquence of this reaction to the body, bio-magnetic circuit will be stalled, resulting in short-circuit. Hence, Dr. Vethathiri has advised aspirants to practice analysis of thoughts in moment to moment awarness as every instance in life is precisely stored in cosmic consicousness and reflected back to you in a course of time. This is called 'Leela' in hindu mythology. Essentially, point here is the diseases could be originated by the karmic influences in you based on what you've accumulated in the past of present. It could be the past karmas based on heriditary. Hence, enlightened masters separated karmas in to two prime categories., one is prarabdha karma, which is the accumulated imprints in yourself based on what you did till date. Wherease, inheritence of the past through genetics is known as sanchita karma. These two karmic influences can drive you crazy. Hence, it is imperative to align yourself with nature through practices of mediation to aleviate sufferings. These are the primary factors of any diseases. The purpose of life is to realize self and align with Nature. Since, you get too attached to the outer, the inner treasures have been forgotton by the mundane mind. You can come back anytime, It's waiting for your return at anymoment like a mom caring her children. Nature is an eternal love and consciousness. It is so precise that anything you did incorrectly against the laws of Nature will have an impact negatively. Hence, you must realize self, study the laws of nature and align yourself to lead a life of over 100 years totally free from diseases in the body. Dr. Vethathiri was a pioneer as he envisaged the dynamics of Mind. He has propagated mind as wave based on his revelations and related to Einstein's theory of relativity. His revelations of the Universe will help Scientists to connect all missing links in particle physics as he declared 'Universe is space' and the 'space is God', thus paved ways to the future scientists and religion to hand shake firmly.

If you're able to analyze your thoughts, then actions can be filtered. For example, If you realize that your boss is bad, then you'd not be reactive despite all humniliations. Hence, a program change is required to your brain cells that to stop being reactive. This is one way to be balanced and remain calm prior to events, whether pleasant or unpleasant. The other way is Vipassana, where in you'd simply observe every moment as taught by the Buddha. Without reacting to the situation, come what may, you'd be objectively observing the situations. This is very unique. Either you'd practice it to subliminate emotions via intellectual reasoning before it occurs as per Dr. Vethathiri or perhaps you can let anything come to your mind, but you'd not react to these situations, regardless of pleasant or unpleasant. There is no other science beyond the above two phenomenon. I have observed these two techniques in my body and the results were amazing. You'll need to practice. For example, at times you'd have reacted to the situation. That's alright, you should remain equanimously and observe. At times, you'd know intellectually a situation is going to be unpleasant, in that case, program your mind to remain calm and composed through reasoning and inquiry.

A lot of your diseases can be stopped using the above techniques. As stated earlier, cumulative desires, pent up emotions results in short-circuits in bio-magnetic body, causing diseases, which can be resolved. The conflict in mind and body can be healed via practices of yoga, meditation, introspection, moment to moment awareness and deep silence once in a while over the weeekend. Your body, mind and soul is an orchestra, which needs some quality time to realize and practices virtual ways of living by aligning with Nature. What can you do if the whole world is polluted by buring fossil fuel?

You can only pray and wish for the welfare of self, family and the society; rest the ultimate Nature will take care. Atleast you can remain calm deeper into super conscious mind and teach your children to love, respect and preserve nature. It is possible to generate fuel, electricity etc without having to destroy nature. You must plant a tree or be part of building a forest to leave a planet for the future.

If your mind is in a constant aggravated state, then it will lead to accelerated condition of cells, thus leading to diseases. Your mind should remain calm where it will help your body rejuvenate itself. The intelligence within your inner self can heal as and when required by liasion with the eternal consciousness. You need to just allow it to work without interrupting it. For example, you must allow enough sleep as required, nutritious food as required, limited work and sex as required. However, anything done in excess will lead to cellular misalignment, thus causing all illness and diseases in the long run. It is imperative to learn ways to align with the ultimate nature. Allopathy has proved to be wrong by only treating the organs. This approach has paralyzed a lot of patients. For example, the one who takes allopathy medications for diabetes will certainly end up with organ failures. A similar story of surgical treatments done cannot help you in anyways unless it is useful for emergency conditions only. For example, cancer cannot be cured in allopathy. It has to allow body to rejuvenate by itself.

Dr. Vethathiri has clearly stated the benefits of aligning with Nature. As a matter of fact, mind, body is so subtle and connected with Nature. Even if you think of doing something bad, it has a ripple effects in mind, and its lineage to the cosmic consciuosness. Hence, everything acts as per laws of Nature. If you do good, you'd reap up the benefits. It's a simple science. What you sow in body, mind is what you'd reap up. For example, If you'd love people, then you'd get love in your life. If you'd sow hate, you'd reap hate. This is based on the revelations of Dr. Vethathiri. Hence, diseases are primarily based on the harmful thinking that is poisoning body, mind genetics and imprints in cosmic consciousness. It will eventually come back to you as effects. The cause and effect of the natural system is very subtle. If you spoil the rhythm by wrong doing, you'd reap up the effects. If you're treating only the effects as diseases, won't help you much.

The meditation practices will increase the energy by liasing mind with the super consiousness, hence there will be an increased state of energy absorbed by the body cells. When your mind is in the mental freuquency of alpha, theta and delta, you're getting closer to the super consiousness, which is the zeroth state as void. As you're able to lower the mental frequency of mind, it will open up pores of mind to absorb cosmic energy. Hence, there will be an incredible rise in the energy levels, which can be harnessed sensibly using introspection to eliminate six temporamental moods and past conditioning.

Further, Dr. Vethathiri's practices involve massage, acupressure and shanthi which are very unique and help in streamlining the third layer of the body, which is the magnetic body. None has analyzed it so far in the medical history, as he was able to realize it as inner revelations by analyzing his whole body. He said: 'Body is a wonder and it mimics the entire Natural phenomenon' and there is no where to go to analyze the principles of nature, except the inner core of the body itself. One of his techniques of introspection involves analysis of thoughts, desires to eliminate mental toxins by removing all conditioning. The emotioal well being is absolutely critical to maintain good health as discussed elaborately in the previous sections. Unless you streamline thoughts, emotions, your energy will be constantly dissipated below the minimum critical level. Just hope and wish for good mentally in meditation. It will yield good results by the law of nature. It is eternal love, and graceful.

As an aspirant progresses to the next stage, he would be able to analyze '*Who am I?*' to realize his self as the manifestations of Nature. Even Buddha mentioned it as '*Asuya*' the chemical reactions in the body causing toxins. Hence, Vipassana plays an important role in aleviating from the conditioning by a simple phenomenon called 'Witnessing'. Come what may, you'd remain calm and witness it. Eventually, all your conditioning will vanish, resulting in deep harmony with oneself. These are the revelations of great englightened masters in India. I can name many more, Osho Rajnessh who had spent his whole life in teaching hundreds of techniques to eliminate conditioning and toxins in body, mind. Dr. Vethathiri's kundalini practices are powerful ways to eliminate toxins. As stated by Maharishi, your astral and causal body is connected to the universal consciousness. It can heal, if you're able to align.

From time memorial, Asian Indians have constructed several temples with mooladhar which indicates cumulative cosmic energy and the one who is deficient of energy can gain benefits by visiting the temples. The plate underneath the main god idol is a made of copper, it can store positive energy and reflect for centuries. Hence, those are deficient in energy levels can regenarate by simply visiting such temples in India. In Auroville, Pondicherry they have created a gigantic structure to harness the energy from sun. The crystal ball stores energy of the sun and reflects. Similarly, there are over thousands of temples in India. These temples were built with a tower kind of structure, for example, Pyramids are all good source of energy. Dr. Patriji of Pyramid Foundation has proved fruits can be stored longer in a pyramid. In essence, these techniques help in restoring energency levels without letting it deplete.

Food is essential. However, it should be taken like medicine in required quantities, with nutritious food which is primarily vegetarian. If you consume animal food, it will result in accumulating toxins in the body. For example, animals do release harmones due to excited state of being before it dies. Hence, these harmones will result in formation of extreme toxic metals in the body and poisonous. Moreso, mental frequency will be aggravated by consumption of alcohol, meat, smoke etc. Dr. Wilson has not anlayzed the above artifacts of vegetarian diet in detail by considering the astral and casual layers of the body. Hence, his analysis was primarily physiology, thus analyzed the chemical properties of changes in the cellular structure. It is imperative to analyze all three layers of body for a complete wellness program, which is missing in Dr. Wilsons nutrition programme, however I'd recommend this program as a good starting point to be aware of food and good habits as you could eventually progress to the next steps of total healing and spiritual progression by combining yoga exercies, meditation and introspection analysis.

I believe disease is simply evidence of the body's whole system out of balance, which is a sort of short circuit in the flow of bio-magnetic energy.

Indeed, the above analogy of Dr.Wilson is true as we realize diseases are prolonged short circuits in the body, mind. A simple stress in mind can perhaps trigger a migraine. When the whole body system becomes balanced and strengthened at root levels, most "disease entities" disappear on their own without a need to know all about them and without a need to name them. A disease can be induced by the past karmas from the genetics too. It is possible. The only way to treat is by constant liaison with nature and not just the diet.

The above analogy is similar to that of Siddhic tradition of India, however with the differences in using herbs for healing. For example, if someone is diseased, his biochemistry is skewed with less resistence. Hence, they had used herb medicines to restore biomagnetic circuit in the body, mind which is totally organic. There was no side effect, here is where allopathy seem to have changed our perceptions by abruptly repressing diseases in the body, instead of healing it organically. Our glands and organs are being suppressed in allopathy, causing long term illness. It's good for short term remedies such as treating cut or wounds or surgical methods for emergency such as accidents.

I am in complete agreement with Dr.Wilson regarding his findings of allopathy that is harming the body. Allopathy is a danger and it has not cured diabetis, thyroid, asthma etc. It is good for treating cuts or wounds and not suitable for treating diseases holistically. I don't believe mostly complex surgeries do help in rejuvenating body. Indeed, many surgeries have resulted in various other complications and other issues, since it is not treated holistically. In my view, surger should be the last option if all other alternate therapies fail.

These diseases simply indicates a certain chemical reaction in the body as a result of alergic reaction, which can be healed by identifying the root causes. Hence, by using methods such as nutritional balancing, it is possible to totally heal your self. I'd even recommend any other alternate methods other than allopathy can certainly help with no long term side effects. I am certain, nutritional balancing is unique with its approach to allow body to heal naturally. Probably, you can adapt this method at an early age to live longer, healthier free from diseases. However, I am surprised Dr. Wilson has not analyzed the critical factors of mind, which is one of the root causes of all diseases in the body. These conflicts form critical factors in formation of diseases. Your psyche causes diseases in the body. You cannot treat body in isolation without identifying the root causes in the mind. Mostly, karmic influences play a major role in the diseases as it alters cellular structure causing short circuits in the body.

Hence, I recommend in addition to the nutritional balancing program, you may need to understand karmic influences known as imprints and dynamics of mind that causes chemical reaction in the body, mind. Also, I insist you'r not just the physiology. There is an eternal lineage to the cosmic consciousness linked to your astral and causal layers. Hence, these frequent short-circuits will result in diseases in the body. Mind is wave. My point is to extend nutritional balancing program to the mind analysis and techniques formulated by Indian siddhas to practice meditation & remaining silence in addition to evolve spiritual beyond body. Otherwise, you'll miss the whole point of any wellness programs around the world. Howsoever you eat healthy, you'll not be healed completely as the roots are somewhere else.

Dr. Wilson may not have analyzed holistically as West is primarily analytical. West has limited limitations of mind as a wave. These are the revelations of enlightened masters of the East. Dr. Wison missed out the critical aspects of the astral (life-force/sub-atomic particles) and causal (magnetic) bodies which are layers of body beyond the physiology. Nutritional balacing program is Diet and lifestyle-based. The core of this system of healing depends upon a proper diet and lifestyle. This program suggests eating a lot of cooked vegetables three times daily. Perhaps, this is a very good starting point and motivation to get away from the sedentary life style. Its good way to stop drinking, eating out frequently, munching habits, smoking, alcohol and immoral sexual habits etc. You should extend beyond body to understand your lineage to Nature and evolution into spirituality by aligning with the eternal consciousness.

Nutritional balancing programs always include eight to ten rather simple nutritional supplements to supply basic nutrients. The products usually include a multivitamin specially formulated for one's metabolic type, supplementary calcium, magnesium, zinc, kelp and trimethylglycine. Perhaps a glandular supplement, and in some cases a few others. In my view, all these supplements are fine as long as it is not chemical based, organic is good for health as it will assimilate naturally. However, I believe these supplements are optional, as the nutrition program can handle it entirely with just the vegetarian diet in moderation and the procedures outlined below. In most cases, in a few weeks to a month or so, one will be able to tolerate the supplements better. Dr. Vethathiri has insisted on eating only required quantify of food, leaving space in stomach, which would help you assimilate radiations from isotopes at the centre of earth. These radiations would help your cells absorb required nutrition. All sorts of vitamin deficiencies are due to over-eating without allowing your body to absorb nutrients from atmosphere.

As I've stated in the earlier section, your body has intelligent system to absorb required minerals from the planets, source of energy such as sun, air, water, land & akash etc. This would apply only if you're able to keep your system light with half-stomach filled. I was amazed to read Jasmuheen, who has mentioned about the prana program, which is a way to survive with less food intake, instead she practiced yoga and meditation to absorb nutrients from atmosphere. She has proved that it is possible to live healthy and longer with less than a meal/day. In our case, perhaps we should keep it simple by eating nutritious and organic food with less toxins. Moreover, extreme care should be taken to keep mental health via meditaiton and introspection to avoid karmic influences.

Choosing the supplements and dosing them is done using a special method of interpreting a hair tissue mineral analysis, preferably from hair on the head, face, underarm or chest, and not pubic hair. Hair testing is a mineral biopsy of the body, and completely different than blood and urine tests. Though, urine and blood tests will help in identifying the cause of infections, sugar levels etc, mineral test results will yield more about the health. Perhaps, this is a useful analysis to baseline.

The hair must not be washed at the laboratory and it must be interpreted according to stress theory and cybernetic methods, not others. It is recommended to do hair tests in analytical Research Labs, because most of these labs do not do the test properly and results are not accurate enough. I don't think this test is available in many other countries as I have realized limited resources in India and many Asian countries.

The hair test is repeated every 3 to 6 months to monitor progress, and to change the nutritional balancing program in order to keep the body chemistry properly balanced as it heals. This is also critical for the success of the programs. At times, one must change the program before it is time for a retest of the hair. Now, let's take a look at de-toxification procedures. I am not sure how far these tests yield accurate metabolic routine as your body is not just chemical properties alone. There is a magnetic circuit aligned with the cosmic consciousness. If you're connected with the cosmos, the universe will heal you internally including the chemical properties of body as simply it is an appropriate ratio of land:air:water:fire: akash aka energy particles etc. If these five elements are balanced, then it is possible to control the chemical reaction. I don't believe Dr. Watson has analyzed this ratio of five core elements. If you carefully examine Cu for example, it looks like this:

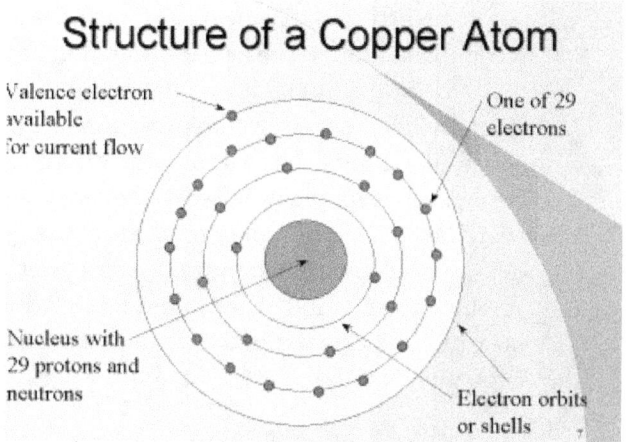

Structure of a Copper Atom

Valence electron available for current flow

One of 29 electrons

Nucleus with 29 protons and neutrons

Electron orbits or shells

The above figure illustrates structure of Copper atom. I was trying to analyze how these electrons are causing toxic chemical reaction in the body. These electrons are tagged to the nucleus via magnetic energy dervied by the electros and the cosmic gravitation force that binds them together. I believe the natural cosmic energy would reduce the toxicity by aligning the atomic structure of Cu or the cellular structure in the body. Either way it would perhaps align it to reduce toxic chemical reaction in the body. I am not saying toxic metals such as mercury, aluminium, lead and cadmium does not cause harm to the body. It does increase your oxidative stress and may trigger medical conditions . Perhaps, not all these metals in the body cause similar chemical reaction as that of consumed as poison for instance. Hence, it is good to realize the value of detox procedures and combine along with yoga, meditation etc.

Nutritional balancing also includes a recommendation to use a near infrared light sauna for detoxification of body. Another highly recommended detoxification procedure are daily coffee enemas or even a simple water enema. I'd rather keep it simple by sun bathing, brisk walking everyday and simple water or oil enema as my objectives are simplified nutritional program combined with mind analysis and remediation measures to heal your body, mind in totality and align with Nature.

You must keep your body light to practice yoga and meditation better. Primarily, your digestive system, lungs should be clear to be able to practice deep meditation. In SKY yoga practices, there are

simple practices taught that would help you keep a
good spine by practicing makarasana, simplified
breating practices such as kabalapathi to remove
toxins in lungs. Also, exercies should be done as
prescribed to ensure stress build in muscles are
relieved by using postures. In fact, kriyas such as
'Sudharshan Kriya', taught by Sri Sri Ravi Shankar,
Art of Living, Vasi Yoga are all powerful ways to
eliminate mental stress that causes toxins in the body.
For example, sudharshan kriya is a powerful
technique to de-condition your body, mind from
stress related ailments. I have observed significant
changes post intensive kriya. It refreshes your whole
body, mind with high energy levels by retrieving
prana energy from the cosmos. A simle Ana pana of
the Buddha can be powerful if practiced diligently
over a period of time. If you like bhajans, songs, It's
a good way to detoxification of mind. The entire
ancient Asia-India portrayed classical art and
architecture such as Bharat Natya, Kathak, Kalari and
many other techniques portrayed cultural evolution
of Indians aligned with Nature.

The objectives of Dr. Vethathiri's SKY yoga
program is to keep a healthy body, mind and
spiritual progression by streamlining air, heat, air,
bio-magnetic energy and blood circulation in the
body. The SKY practices combines mental analysis to
eliminate conditioning at the roots, thus alieviating
diseases at its root.

For example, six temporamental moods such
as greed, anger, immoral sexual passion, vanity and

vengeance. Each of it causes mental stress and alters cellular structure to create toxins in the body. The very moment a thought is induced in brain cells will invoke a certain chemical reaction in the body, mind causing disruption of bio-magnetic flow. Similarly, anything that you do the environment externally will impact. For example, if you deforest, then you'd face an ecological disaster. The West has equivocally used chemical fertilizers, thus causing an ecological disaster. The entire agriculture is in jeopardy due to extensive usage of fertilizers such as urea, dioxin chemical fertilizers. A similar act by allopathic doctors using antibiotics is causing a disaster in your body, which is losing its inherent potential. West has not analyzed holistically. It has killed your natural antibiotics in the body, and micro organisms in land causing ecological disaster. It is imperative for the people of the World to realize these harmful effects.

This can be aleviated by practices meditation and sublimation techniques. Its not good enough, as deeper state of silence will yield a lot of karmic patters escalating from the deeper core of sub-conscious and un-conscious mind. These strands stored as magnetic strips in cells as DNA must be sublimated by the way of deeper analysis and sublimation techniques like super-imposition and/or witnessing or combining either of these approaches to detoxify mind. Mind and body are inter-related, without treating at the grass roots, you cannot aleviate yourself from pain and miseries.

Unless you sit in deeper state of meditation, you cannot detoxify mind, body. I mean detoxifying mind is an essential process of cleansing all karmic patterns in the mind. Each of these karmic patterns could have originated from this birth or perhaps inherited through genetics. It is registered as DNA strands in brain cells, body cells and organs. Hence, it is imperative to heal the karmic patterns by liaison with the cosmic consciousness. By frequently dipping in the super consciousness, you'll be able to dissolve all karmic patterns. It gets nullified, however you should not invoke the behavior again.

A deeper practices of meditation and remaining silent in deeper state of consciouses can easily wipe out all your karmic patterns. You'll be able to remain calm naturally without any efforts. It will re-align your cells. These aspects were not discussed in the nutritional program by Dr. Wilson, as he may not have explored the other dimension of mind beyond just the body.

Dr. Vethathiri has combined acupressure and foot reflexology, which are amazing and simple healing method. One can do it at home on oneself, or another person can assist. Another recommended procedure is 'Makarasana' to twist the spine daily to help keep the spine loose and correct some subluxations of the spine. The SKY practices has acupressure, foot refloxogy, hand, leg exercises and massage to ensure blood, air, heat and bio-magnetic circulation is streamlined. The above physical exercises are covered as part of any yoga regime in simplified kundalini yoga or any other hatha yoga practices, surya namashkar etc. However, you must consult a good yoga practitioner before practicing any exercies. For example, sirash asana (upside down) is very dangerous. Be aware, as this sirash asana is not good. Also, if you take homeopathy or any other alternate medicines, please checkout the credibility with necessary certifications. yoga/meditation is not new for India, may be new for the United States of America. These are known as makarasana practices, intended for keeping your spine healthy.

Finally, all of these together constitute the procedures of nutritional balancing combined with yoga practices to heal body, mind and take your soul to the eternity. They are not required, but they speed progress and are essential for some people in order to become healthy. The above technique is part of any yoga program. You may explore 'Simplified Kundali Yoga (SKY) founded by Maharishi Vethathiri and Vipassana founded by The Buddha' operating worldwide, that teaches holistic physical exercises and meditation. Vipassana is a wonderful technique over 2000 years to aleviate you from the deepest core of conditioning in the sub-conscious and unconscious layers of mind. A lot of pent-up emotions are held in the deepest core of mind as untreated. Whenver there is a right opportunity, it may escalate to the conscious mind. These exercises are unique as it will alter the cellular patterns and help in dissolving karmic patterns, which is the real detoxification of body, mind. I insist Dr. Wilson to explore this technique to realize the values of mind and elevating soul towards eternity.

Also, the unique kaya kalpa practices formulated by Dr. Maharishi Vethathiri helps in rejuvenation of sexual vital fluid as it is like a battery supplying energy particles throughout the body. The quality and quantity of sexual vital fluid results in a sound body, mind. If it is diluted, then it will result in all sorts of diseases. Perhaps, Dr. Wilson was not even aware of sexual vital fluid and its benefits beyond sensory pleasures. These are deeply ingrained in the wisdom of eastern mystics. You must practice witnessing situations, without getting bogged down by the events happening aroud you. This is a unique practices of Vipassana, formulated by the Buddha. Let's take a quick look at the history of nutritional balancing science.

HISTORY OF NUTRITIONAL BALANCING SCIENCE

From time immorial, Asian-Indian siddhas have tried keeping body, mind healthy. However, their objectives were just not the disease free body, instead to extend life to realize self by liasion with the ultimate Nature. They have found have unique techniques to cleanse body, and heal by itself. However, their strategy was a holistic method and not treating the respective organs alone by analyzing the root causes. Similarly, these methods included techniques to use herbs, natural medicines from roots, leaves without harming the body. It helped in boosting the immune, until the natural immunity is restory.

The Nutritional balancing science of the 19th century was developed by Dr. Paul C. Eck, during the late 1970s and early 1980s. Dr. Eck was a mineral researcher who spent his entire adult life developing the ideas and practical application of this science.

With nutritional balancing, healing of symptoms takes place at its own pace, and in its own order. This is quite different than remedy sciences such as drug medicine, herbs, homeopathy and most naturopathy. I believe Dr. Wilson has not analyzed the benefits of herbs, or any other alternate medicines. These are all organic and in my view they just induce your body to produce antibiotics organically, hence there is no side effect of medicines using herbs, homeopathy etc. Now, let's understand the concept of retracing, which is going back in memory to treat your mind. I personally found it very useful, however this technique of retracing should be done very carefully as you should be practicing awareness. I practiced Vipassana to be able to retrace without any efforts at all. The results were just amazing and all your past wounds would heal one after the other.

These are called retracings, a concept that is well known in chiropractic, but not in allopathic medical science. It only occurs with deep healing programs, of which nutritional balancing or Vipassana or Dr. Vethathiri's SKY deep silence program, where you'd allow your sub-conscious imprints to surface to the conscious state of mind.

The Nutritional balancing programs involve some discipline and commitment of time and energy to learn and follow the diet, take the supplements, and hopefully to do the procedures.

The primary difference between organic compounds and inorganic compounds is that organic compounds always contain carbon while most inorganic compounds do not contain carbon. Also, almost all organic compounds contain carbon-hydrogen or C-H bonds. Note, *containing carbon is not sufficient* for a compound to be considered organic!. As step 1, you should restrict consumption of inorganic food and non-vegetarian including sea food. This is an exception from the origional nutrition program, however my recommendations is based on combining siddhic tradition. Be conscious of what you eat and eat only when you're hungry and drink only when you feel thirsty. Eat in moderation with satvic food (light vegetarian meal) to remain healthy and for spiritual progression. Hence, you should try and remain with an Organic diet as much as possible.

There are proven side affects of non-vegetarian food due to toxins generated in the animal, which is consumed. Hence, it is the basic attribute that should be avoided. Unfortunately, Dr. Wilson has not analyzed it deep enough to reveal the negative impact of consuming non-vegetarian food. It is a misconception that vegetarian food is less nutritious. It is not mandatory to consume non-vegetarian food to continue with this nutritional balancing program. Now, let's understand Dr. Vethathiri's revelations of body, mind and soul.

There are three layers of body.,
a. Physical layer made up of cells,
b. Astral layer made up of sub-atomic particles aka life-force particles &
c. Causal layer made up of shadow wave particles aka magnetic layer

Dr. Vethathiri has mentioned the second layer and third layers are eternal. Only the physical layer dies and bound by the chemical reactions. These two layers can help in cleansing the whole body if it is wired with the eternal consciousness. It's like connectig your mobile with the global network. Dr.Wilson's research was primarily based on the a. Physical layer only. Hence, it focuses pre-dominantly on the cellular chemical properties and reactions.

However, there is no revelations of b. Astral or c. Casual layer. These layers are intangile layers which governs the physical layer. For example, there is a ratio of 1:100:1000 maintained in proportion to manage a healthy body, mind and soul. As stated by Dr. Maharishi Vethathiri based on his revelations, b. Astral layer and c. Causal layers are formed by the countless billions of sub-atomic particles spinning at a very high velocity. Thus, forming Astral layer, which is turn forms waves due to the spinning sub-atomic particles. It's like a ripple wave. Thus, it forms astral and causal layers.

These ratio of physical:astral: casual should be maintained in right proportion. For example, if you're subjected to emotional state such as anxiety, stress or anger, this condition will excite the layer b, and c which are proportionately aggravated. In the above analogy, astral layer comprising of countless billions of spinning sub-atomic particles at a velocity of say 10 metre/sec, will be subjected to 100 metre/sec velocity. This accelerated state will subject your causal body to expand in volume, meaning the shadow waves emanated by these countless billions of sub-atomic particles would form a wave length pattern from 100 nanometres/sec to 500 nanometres/sec.

This would result in increased volume and the energy loss/second in the body would be higher than the energy produced in the body. Now, this would result in cellular structure taking the request for increased production to meet the shortage. This analogy is similar to the increased energy production from the transmission line, hence the production generator has to be cranck in more energy than usual, thus resulting in reduced life cycle term of the engine. This holds good for the cellular structure as well. Due to your emotional reaction in the mind, would result in the increased request for cells to spin more aggressively to meet the production line requirements.

Thus, phsyical:astral:casual layers will be subjected to enormous misalignment. Any thought induced in mind has an impact to the physique, these thoughts invoked via brain cells create an environment in body, which may be pleasant or unpleasant. For example, an emotion of the past such as job loss could trigger unplesant situation in body, mind, thus causing chemical reaction in the body. This would impact your flow of blood, air, heat and bio-magnetic circulation. This is the epitome of Dr. Vethathiri's SKY technique as well as the Buddha's Vipassana. In Vipassana, you'd learn how to remain equinanimously despite external and internal stimuli by simply witnessing the situation without reacting to it. The same analogy holds true for SKY practices if you do it correctly by practicing non-reactiveness despite the situation. Eventually, it would help you restore a lot of energy to keep your harmonal balances and bio-magnetic reserves to boost your immune levels.

Thus, many enlightened souls were able to heal any diseased. It was possible due to huge reservoir of energy stored in their body. It is possible for you, if you'd practice yoga, meditation diligently as a daily routine. You can remain free of stress in mind and diseases in the body. As per Dr. Vethathiri, the significance of karmic influences in the body would show up as diseases in the body and conflicts in mind. Hence, it is imperative to treat body, mind at grass root levels, instead of just the body.

Next point is the sexual vital fluid, which produces countless billions of sub-atomic particles like a battery. If it is diluted, intensity of sub-atomic particles would reduce, thus resulting in exposing body to diseases. Therefore, extreme caution and responsiveness is required in maintaining proper sex health in moderation. Excess would result in dissipated fluids, thus resulting in reduced sub-atomic particles generated. Moreover, it will expose your cells to diseases in the long run.

Now, imagine the number of times that you're subjected to emotional stress causing distress in the body. So, nutrional balancing combined with mind analysis and sublimation of karmic influences would result in longetivity of life –span without diseases.

Dr. Vethathiri has mentioned about food that is convered to juice, blood, flesh, fat, bone, bone marrow and sexual vital fluid. Body needs proteins, vitamins, carbohydrates and minerals for energy. However, food is not the only source of energy as stated earlier. There are other sources such as air, water, radiations from other planets and sun. Your body is so delicatly connected to Nature and there has been no separation, except your greedy mind. Generally, yoga and meditaiton practices will regulate your glands since the focus on breadth or kunadlini will regulate all glands. Hencec, there is no separate program required for regulating harmone levels and wbc in blood. It will be rejuventated by practicing kaya kalpa exercise.

What is that you've achieved by letting your mind wander and wander for years since you were a teenager? It's been a futile exercise in seeking pleasures in mundane activities. Mind is intended to expand to eternity and your natural desire is to become eternal. Dr. Vethathiri has clearly mentioned whatsoever you do, whatsoever you achieve in mundane world cannot fulfill you as you're really seeking something eternal. That something eternal is within you and outside you. This is called 'Unified Force', god or love or nature. Unless you're liaising with nature, you'd never feel contended despite having the most beautiful lady beside you, all the wealth in the world, BMW's or Benz etc. etc. Nothing can satisfy you as you're seeking eternal being which is the source of you. While you need to detoxify body, it is essential to detoxifying mind. The act of detoxifying body is yoga exercises and the act of detoxifying mind is meditation and introspection. You'd be able to achieve primal concsiousness, the purest state of your own being.

I believe if you allow Nature, it will detoxify your body, mind. The "I" (Ego) must dissolve into the super consciousness in deeper state of consciousness to align with Nature. With love and compassion it is possible to heal quicker. Mostly 90% of issues are mind related, hence it is possible to heal totally using the above practices. Primarily, yoga practices focus on cleansing body by cleansing glands, removing toxins, lungs clearanc, digestive tracks and colon clearance with spinal cord clearance.

It also works holistically in all three layers by streamlining flow of sub-atomic partices in the body and magnetic flow in mind. Since, mind is wave, a reduced frequency will lead to connecting your micro-soul to macro-soul. Hence, the de-toxification process happens at deeper levels.

In the next chapter, let us take a deep dive of hair mineral test analysis.

***

Chapter 2

Hair Mineral Analysis

The hair mineral test analysis reveals mineral deficiencies and heavy metal toxicity. But many people don't realize that it also provides a blueprint to increase your performance, improve energy. Hair mineral analysis reveals and explains the causes of many health symptoms and disease, whose underlying causes are largely related to nutritional deficiencies, mineral imbalances and heavy metal and chemical toxicity.

Your hair can be tested because it is one of many places the body eliminates minerals and heavy metals. The individual mineral levels, ratios of minerals to each other and patterns of minerals deposited in the hair reveal all kinds of things about your body chemistry and health conditions.

Unlocking Human Performance

Your physical and cognitive abilities can be optimized using hair tissue mineral analysis (HTMA). The nutrient mineral levels and their comparative relationships (ratios) determine how well your cells function and impact physical and cognitive performance. The goal is to correct body chemistry and improve cell functioning using HTMA as a guide for targeted supplementation.

The problem is that when you are *tired,* you might use a stimulant like an energy drink. If we are too *wired* we might use a sedative, alcohol, or another drug to relax. We are smart enough to realize that these substances affect our biochemistry, but they instead create biochemical chaos. Misguided biochemistry balancing leads to all types of undesirable health consequences.

This is why it's so much better to balance biochemistry intelligently using hair mineral analysis. Intelligent biochemical balancing using Mineral Power which utilizes HTMA, is simply about eating a nutrient-rich diet, targeted nutrient supplement therapy, detoxification and learning to avoid things that cause you harm. Benefits include improved cognitive function, more energy, correcting the metabolic rate (weight loss), emotional stability and greater stress resilience.

Individuals at the leading edge of intellectual and physical performance, including CEO's, professional athletes, high-level entertainers, elite military, top scientists, and intellectuals, know the value of excellent nutrition and its positive effect on performance. By improving your nutritional status and balancing biochemistry with HTMA, you will experience a higher state of performance.

What Can a Hair Mineral Analysis reveal?

The hair mineral analyses are screening tests only and do not diagnose disease. Perhaps, you can combine with blood and urine tests if you suspect any diseases in the body. However, a properly interpreted hair analysis can reveal various mineral imbalances that indicate a tendency for various conditions. A hair mineral analysis provides a picture of body chemistry including:

1. Heavy Metal Toxicity
2. Mineral Deficiencies and Imbalances
3. Metabolic Rate (fast or slow)
4. Adrenal Fatigue
5. Thyroid Function
6. Nervous System Imbalances
7. Protein Synthesis
8. Inflammation
9. Energy Levels
10. Mental Health Issues
11. Liver & Kidney Stress
12. Carbohydrate Tolerance &
13. Blood Sugar Imbalances like Diabetes and Insulin resistance

Why Test for Minerals?

Minerals are the "spark plugs" of life. They are involved in almost all enzyme reactions in the body. Without enzyme activity, life does not exist. The foundation of health lies in adequate mineral intake and ideal mineral ratios. Anything else you do for your health is great, but minerals must be the foundation and priority. Once those are balanced and replenished, it solves the majority of health issues people attempt in vain to correct by other means.

The hair analysis graph shows the following nutrient minerals: calcium, magnesium, sodium, potassium, iron, copper, manganese, zinc, chromium, selenium and more. These minerals are necessary for proper functioning of the organs and tissues of the body, but can also metastasize (store in organs where they're not supposed to be) and prevent proper function. Many minerals need to be replenished, while some forms of minerals need to be detoxed if they are forms the body cannot utilize.

Balancing minerals with a hair mineral analysis is imperative to achieve proper mineral ratios. All the minerals have a complex interaction and affect each other. Excess intake of a single mineral can decrease the intestinal absorption of another mineral. For example, a high intake of calcium depresses intestinal zinc absorption, while an excess intake of zinc can depress copper absorption. It is evident that a loss of homeostatic equilibrium between nutrients has an adverse effect upon health.

Common Causes of Mineral Imbalances

Many factors contribute to mineral deficiencies and imbalances. Here are only a few:

- Stress depletes minerals from the body, most notably magnesium and zinc.
- **Toxic Metals and Chemicals.** They can replace minerals in enzyme binding sites and interfere with mineral absorption.
- Chronic viral and bacterial infections are subtle stressors on the body, depleting minerals. Many suffer from gut dysbiosis, Lyme and many other low-grade chronic infections.
- **Toxic Food Supply.** Our food and soils are depleted of minerals, which is why everyone needs nutritional supplements. Hybrid crops, superphosphate fertilizers (i.e. Miracle Grow), refined foods, pesticides, food additives and more, all contribute to a nutritionally depleted and toxic food supply.
- **Drinking Water.** Tap water is not safe due to added chlorine, aluminum, fluoride and sometimes copper, which cause toxicity or displace other minerals.
- **Unhealthy lifestyles.** Many individuals do not get enough sleep, don't exercise enough or have other unhealthy lifestyle habits.

Heavy Metal Toxicity

Presently, humanity is exposed to the highest levels of toxic metals in recorded history, up to several thousand times higher than just a hundred years ago. Everyone has metals in their body; the question is how much do you have? Removing them from the body can vastly improve health, mental functioning, energy and performance.

Hair mineral analysis is a toxicology screen for metals including uranium, lead, mercury, cadmium, arsenic, aluminum and nickel. No test, including urine, stool or blood tests, can show all your heavy metals toxicities as they are buried deep in the bones, brain and organs. Thus, they will not be revealed on a hair tissue test or any other test, until they are mobilized from storage. Only continuous monitoring through any means over a period of years while doing a detox program can reveal all your heavy metal toxicities. In this regard, HTMA is a reliable indicator of toxicity and is helpful in monitoring detoxification progress.

Many health conditions are caused or exacerbated by heavy metal toxicity. Metals can contribute to any imaginable health ailment or condition including cases of diabetes (iron), cancer (cadmium), multiple sclerosis (mercury), Alzheimer's disease (aluminum), and others.

The most common toxicities include:

The copper dysregulation is one of the most commonly encountered imbalances that we find on hair tests and is a contributor to many health problems including cancer, weight gain, eating disorders, fatigue, premenstrual syndrome, endometriosis, fibroids, ovarian cysts, infertility, depression, anxiety, and bipolar disorder, migraine headaches, allergies, ADHD and learning disorders.

Mercury is found in almost everyone from consuming fish, although it's also in the atmosphere as a result of coal burning. Mercury toxicity is associated with countless health issues including adrenal dysfunction, thyroid dysfunction, depression, dizziness, fatigue, headaches, insomnia, gut dysbiosis, kidney damage, memory loss, mood swings, numbness and tingling and muscle weakness.

Aluminum is the most common element of the earth's crust and is a very common toxicity. Aluminum has been found to be associated with Alzheimer's, Parkinson's and other forms of dementia, anemia and other blood disorders, colic, fatigue, and kidney and liver dysfunctions.

How to Balance Minerals

A hair mineral analysis can give you a crystal ball and preview into your state of health because it can show health issues and body chemistry imbalances before you manifest symptoms. Once you present with symptoms or illness like cancer, for instance, you've been sick for many years – even decades. A hair mineral analysis will give you a place to begin and a plan to improve your health beyond what you thought imaginable.

Mineral Power uses hair mineral analysis to address the root causes of physical and mental health issues – nutrient deficiencies and heavy metal and chemical toxicity – and provides a plan to resolve these issues. So many health issues are not resolved with traditional medical care because these issues are rarely addressed.

A Mineral Power program provides you with a diet plan, targeted nutrient therapy, detox protocols like infrared saunas and coffee enemas, and lifestyle recommendations. It is a powerful program proven to reverse disease and improve health symptoms. You can naturally improve your performance, vitality, energy and mental clarity, and truly become Bulletproof.

Hair tissue mineral analysis or HTMA is a soft tissue mineral biopsy that uses hair as the sampling tissue. A biopsy is an analysis of a body tissue. Hair is considered a soft tissue, and hence hair analysis is a soft tissue biopsy. The test measures the levels of 20 or more minerals in the hair with an accuracy of plus or minus about 3%. This is about the same level of accuracy as most blood tests, or a little better. For accurate measurement of the water-soluble elements, the hair sample must not be washed at the hair testing laboratory. The preparation of the hair sample at the laboratory is a debate that exists among the laboratories that offer hair mineral testing. Most laboratories, unfortunately, wash the hair with powerful detergents and toxic solvents such as acetone or alcohol.

As an aside, hair is extremely useful for testing many things besides minerals. These include drugs, toxic chemicals and DNA. These, however, are not the focus of this article. Hair is frequently used in forensic medicine, and in drug testing clinics. It is also used worldwide for biological monitoring of many animal species for toxic metals. It is a measure of the radiance of the body, and of the brain, in particular. This is not easy to explain, but somehow the mineral deposition in the hair tissue reflects the vitality of a human being or animal.

The hair mineral test's ability to assess and predict physical and psychological states of the body is quite unlike blood, urine, feces.

For example, the hair mineral test provides indicators of inflammation, but inflammation can manifest as any of 20 or 30 medical diagnoses. Another example is the hair test can provide information about calcium deposition in the soft tissues. However, calcium deposition can manifest as any of at least 10 or so medical conditions such as arteriosclerosis, arthritis, spondylitis, bursitis, gall stones and more.

History and development of hair mineral testing. Mineral testing by atomic absorption spectroscopy was developed almost 100 years ago. It has been, and continues to be, the standard way to test for minerals in geology, agriculture, plant, animal and human tissue studies. It is also the standard method of environmental mineral testing used throughout the world.

Human hair tissue mineral analysis became widely available in the 1970s. The development of computer-controlled spectrometers advanced the accuracy and reliability of testing, and reduced the cost.

Why measure minerals? Minerals are sometimes called the 'sparkplugs' of the body. They are needed for millions of enzymes as co-factors, facilitators, inhibitors and as part of the enzymes themselves. As a result, minerals have a great deal to do with the health of our bodies. By analyzing mineral imbalances in the body, one can learn a lot about the causes and correction of hundreds of common physical and mental health conditions.

A specific class of minerals, the toxic metals, is also extremely important today due to a nutritionally depleted food supply and the presence of environmental toxicity almost everywhere on planet earth. Studying toxic metals is thus very important today to monitor their spread and learn about their many damaging effects upon the bodies of human beings, animals, plants and other organisms.

Even more can be learned about human and animal health by studying the ratios of the major minerals in the body. This is a more complex area, but a very important and fruitful one. Finally, by studying more complex patterns of minerals in the body, one can learn even more about human health and disease.

I believe hair makes an excellent testing material for many reasons:

1. the most important reason is that it works for nutritional balancing assessment.

2. Simple and non-invasive. Sampling is simple and non-invasive.

3. A stable biopsy material. Hair is a stable biopsy material that remains viable for years, if needed. It also requires no special handling, and can be mailed easily.

4. Easy to measure mineral levels. Mineral levels in the hair are about ten times that of blood, making them easy to detect and measure accurately in the hair.

5. Rapidly growing tissue. Hair is a fairly rapidly growing tissue. This enables one to obtain a recent biochemical picture of soft tissue metabolism.

6. A non-essential, excretory tissue. The body often throws off toxic substances in the hair, since the hair will be cut off and lost to the body. This is very helpful to identify toxic metals, for example, and other things.

7. Wide variation in the readings. Mineral levels are kept relatively constant in the blood, even when pathology is present. This must be done because blood touches all the body tissues, and too much variation is dangerous. This is the reason many people have normal blood tests even when they are quite ill.

Hair minerals do not circulate, and pose no threat to the body. Values often vary by a factor of ten or much more, making measurement easier and providing a tremendous amount of accurate knowledge about the cells and the soft tissue of our bodies.

8. Easier detection of toxic metals - Toxic metals are easier to detect in the hair than in the blood. The body quickly removes toxic metals from the blood, if it can. For this reason, most toxic metals are not found in high concentrations in the blood, except right after an acute exposure.

In contrast, many toxic metals accumulate in the soft tissues such as the hair because the body tries to move them to locations where they will do less damage. Hair testing provides a long-term reading, while blood tests and urine tests provide a more in-stantaneous reading of the body. Both types of read-ings have value. For example, blood tests can vary from minute to minute, depending upon one's diet, activities, the time of day and many other factors. This is beneficial in some instances, but is often less helpful when seeking an overall metabolic reading. At this time, (2016) blood tests do not work for nutri-tional balancing assessment.

Cost-effective, accurate and reliable - Ad-vancements in computer-controlled mass spectrosco-py and other technologies have rendered the hair mineral biopsy an extremely cost-effective, accurate and reliable test when it is performed well. The US federal government licenses all hair mineral testing labs in this nation, and similar programs assure quality in other nations, as well.

WHAT DOES THE HAIR MINERAL TEST MEASURE?

The test only measures minerals. They are locked into the hair as it grows. One can assess:

1. Mineral levels. These are the actual numbers or readings of the minerals on the test.

2. Mineral ratios. This adds significant complexity and a great deal more information. Dr. Paul Eck found that the ratios are usually more important than the levels of the minerals. This has to do with homeostatic states of body chemistry, which means states of balance or equilibrium. These are represented by ratios between the minerals.

3. Simple patterns. These are combinations of the levels and/or ratios.

4. Complex patterns. These consist of combinations of levels, ratios and simple patterns.

5. Changes over time and the rate of change. By comparing two or more tests when a person has followed a nutritional balancing program, one can discern changes over time of the levels, ratios, simple patterns and complex patterns. One can also discern the rate of change of all these.

Which minerals are tested? The hair test provides a measure of the chemical elements deposited in the cells and between the cells of the hair. It provides a reading of the deposition of the mineral in the hair during the 3-4 months during which the hair grew. It does not measure the total body load of any mineral, as some claim.

At least 20 elements are measured, depending on the laboratory. The three groups of elements tested are:

1. Macro-minerals include calcium, magnesium, sodium, potassium and phosphorus. Some labs also read sulfur.

2. Trace Minerals include iron, zinc, copper, manganese, selenium, chromium, and some labs measure others.

3. Toxic Minerals include lead, mercury, cadmium, arsenic, aluminum, and nickel. Some labs read others as well. Toxic metals are discussed at length in a separate article entitled Toxic Metals.

How are the readings reported? The mineral values are usually reported in three ways:

1. Milligrams per 100 grams, often written as mg%. This is how Analytical Research Labs reports the numbers.

2. Micrograms per gram or ug/g. This gives numbers that are 10 times higher than milligrams per hundred grams or mg%. To convert the reading to mg%, simply move the decimal point one space to the left. For example, if calcium is reported as 1210 ug/g, it is the same as 121 mg%

3. Parts per million or ppm. This method gives the same numbers as when they are reported in ug/g.

HOW IS HAIR MINERAL TESTING USED BY DOCTORS?

Doctors and nutritionists use the hair mineral test in one of six ways:

Toxic metal testing only - Among the doctors and nutritionists who use mineral testing, most only use it for the detection of high levels of toxic metals. This is one of the least important uses for it, however, from the perspective of nutritional balancing science. Also, hair testing is not that accurate for the detection of all toxic metals in the body.

Replacement therapy of nutrient minerals. A small number of doctors use the hair mineral test to detect low levels of nutrient minerals. Then, most of them suggest replacement therapy. This means that they suggest foods or food supplements to raise the levels of the trace minerals that are low, or lower the ones that are high.

WHAT CAN A MINERAL ANALYSIS REVEAL?

Analyzing hair tissue for chemical elements is quite different from testing blood, urine or feces, although all have great value in the right situation. Hair mineral analysis can reveal the following:

1. Lifestyle imbalances. The test can reveal that a problem in a person's lifestyle - such as drug use, a very unhappy relationship, or a work problem – is impacting the person's health. This is extremely useful, in some cases.

In addition, the test often reveals the highly toxic effects of cigarette and marijuana use (cadmium). It also reveals the toxic effects of body care products such as selenium-containing shampoo, aluminum-containing anti-perspirants, and lead-containing hair dyes.

It may also reveal the toxic effects of medical drugs such as Flonase (antimony), anti-acids (aluminum), and some diuretics (mercury). It can also sometimes reveal occupational or other exposure to toxins such as excess exposure to iron, copper, or manganese in those who work in these industries.

2. Dietary problems. The test contains a number of indicators to help a practitioner discern that a person's diet is inadequate or imbalanced. These include indicators for low protein intake (low phosphorus in some cases), excessive carbohydrate

intake, some drinking water problems, and problems with vegetarian and vegan diets. In addition, the test can identify several foods that contain toxins such as Rooibos tea (nickel and lead toxicity) or eating fish (high in mercury).

3. The metabolic type - This is an important fact of body chemistry. It is most helpful to understand hundreds of symptoms, and to guide the dietary and supplement recommendations. It also helps to understand many emotional and mental symptoms as well.

4. The energy and vitality level - Energy is a common denominator of health. This means that if one's energy is low, hundreds of symptoms can occur. Restoring one's biochemical or adaptive energy is a key to healing. This is one of the most basic of healing principles. A properly interpreted hair mineral analysis is an excellent way to evaluate a person's adaptive energy level, as well as to figure out how to correct it. Also, enough care should be taken to practice meditation, yoga exercises with streamlined thoughts to increase vitality level.

5. Gland and organ activity - Hair mineral testing can provide a number of indicators for the cellular effect of the thyroid and adrenal hormones, and at times the ovarian hormones as well. It can also be used indirectly to assess the activity of the liver, kidneys, stomach, intestines and perhaps other organs as well.

6. Carbohydrate tolerance - The test can quickly screen for hypoglycemia and, at times, diabetes, although a glucose tolerance test (GTT) should be done if one suspects diabetes. Hair testing can, however, usually guide a practitioner to correct Type 2 diabetes and some Type 1 diabetes without the need for most drugs. Mineral imbalances and chronic infections are often involved with these conditions.

7. Toxic metal assessment - No method of testing can detect all the toxic metals in the body because most of them are hidden deep in the body organs and glands. When interpreted properly, however, a hair mineral analysis is often helpful to assess the general level of toxic metals in the body.

8. Trends or tendencies for over 60 common health conditions. This is an amazing benefit. Research indicates that many health conditions are related to tissue mineral imbalances. The test may reveal them months or years before they manifest in the body. This makes possible a powerful preventive medical science. This is much less costly and more effective than waiting until a disease such as cancer or heart disease occurs.

This aspect of hair mineral testing alone would save billions of dollars if it were used widely. For example, one can inexpensively and accurately screen for tendencies for diabetes, heart disease, chronic fatigue, cancer, yeast infections, and many other health conditions.

10. Monitoring Progress. Hair mineral analysis is often helpful to monitor a person's progress on a healing program of any kind. Symptomatic changes alone are often not a good way to know if a person is progressing on a healing program. However, the hair test will often detect subtle changes in body chemistry, another wonderful benefit of this test.

11. Stress patterns. A properly performed hair mineral analysis is superb to assess the stage of stress, as well as 30 or more stress response patterns of the human body.

This type of analysis and interpretation is based on the stress theory of disease, a modern understanding of health and disease.

12. Autonomic nervous system assessment. A properly performed hair mineral test can assess and guide the correction of the activity of the autonomic nervous system.

Problems with this nervous system are very widespread today, and can cause hundreds of symptoms from digestive disturbance and inability to eliminate toxic metals, to sleep disturbances, blood sugar problems and even cancers. Few in the medical, holistic or naturopathic professions know how to address these issues.

13. Psychological/emotional assessment. One the most exciting uses of the hair mineral analysis is the assessment of causes for conditions such as de-

pression, anxiety, panic attacks, attention deficit, brain fog, autism, schizophrenia, dementia, violence, and bipolar disorder. Hair mineral testing often shows why these conditions occur, and how to correct them at a deep level.

14. Trauma. Hair mineral testing can also reveal sociological issues such as some traumas, abuse, and criminality. For more on this topic, please read Trauma Release on this site.

16. Agriculture. The common soil analysis farmer's use is identical to the hair mineral analysis. The principles of nutritional balancing science can be used to help balance the soil and improve crop yield and nutritional quality of our food supply. For more on this topic, please read rejuvenating the Soil with Nutritional Balancing on this site.

17. Other. More is possible with hair mineral testing. One of the most interesting is identifying movement patterns. These have to do with a person's lifestyle and current activities, in relation to the person's life path or progress through life. This can be extremely helpful in counseling a person, and to understand illness, both physical and emotional.

Deep insights into biochemistry, physiology, psychology, pathology and possibly more esoteric sciences, such as biological transmutation of the elements, are also possible using the hair mineral test. Some of these are briefly discussed in the article entitled The Theory of Nutritional Balancing Science.

CURRENT IDEAL HAIR MINERAL VALUES

1. Hair must not be washed at the laboratory for accurate readings.

2. Levels below the ideals listed above generally indicate a poor eliminator of this metal. This is an important concept for hair analysis interpretation. For more on this topic, please read the article entitled Poor Eliminator Pattern on this website.

3. Most people have too much of most of the toxic metals, even if they are not revealed on the test. They can be hidden, sequestered deep within the body tissues. This is especially true of mercury and aluminum, due to environmental contamination.

***

Chapter 3

Toxic Metal &
Detoxification

$\mathbf{T}$oxic metals are a group of minerals that have no known function in the body. In addition, they are known to be very harmful to plant, animal and human bodies. High exposure - Toxic metals have always been present on earth. However, mankind today is exposed to the highest levels of these metals in recorded history. This is mainly due to their industrial use for the past 300 years, the burning of fossil fuels without scrubbers, and improper incineration of waste materials worldwide.

Toxic metals are now everywhere, and affect everyone on planet earth. They have become a major cause of illness, aging and even genetic defects.

Not taught much. The study of toxic metals is often considered a part of the study of toxicology. This subject matter is not widely taught today in high schools, colleges or medical schools. For this reason, this important cause of disease is given little attention in society or in conventional mainstream medicine. Fortunately, environmental science is beginning to pay more attention to toxic metals and their relationship to the health of all living things on planet earth. Let's explore extent of toxic metal problems, sources of toxic metals, symptoms, and how to remove them safely and deeply.

TOXIC METAL CONCEPTS

Let's explore the following principles or concepts about toxic metals.

1. Congenital toxic metals. ALL babies born today anywhere in the world have too many toxic metals. This occurs because toxic metals are widely distributed in the air, drinking water, food and elsewhere.

Also, all the toxic metals pass easily across the placenta from pregnant mothers and deposit in the tissues of their unborn babies. This is a very serious problem that few talk about. However, it is obvious if one does hair mineral testing on newborns and young children.

2. Preferred minerals. The body takes the best minerals it can find from food, water and isotopes. Even the highly toxic ones can sustain life, to a degree. However, our bodies definitely prefer the ideal or nutrient minerals in enzymes and elsewhere, if they can get them.

For example, the body prefers zinc for over 50 critical enzymes. However, if zinc becomes deficient, which it is in most soil and in most of our food today, or if exposure to cadmium, lead or mercury is sufficiently high, the body will use the toxic metals in place of zinc. This can be eliminated by occasional fasting as required to absorb minerals in the atmosphere.

Cadmium, in particular, is located just below zinc in the periodic table of the elements, so its outer atomic structure is very similar to that of zinc. As a result, cadmium "fits" well into zinc binding sites and can easily replace zinc in critical enzymes such as RNA transferee, carboxypeptidase, alcohol dehydrogenase and many others of great importance in the body.

An analogy is to imagine taking an automobile journey. If one is far away from a repair shop when a key part such as the fan belt breaks, if one had a spare piece of rope, one could tie it around the pulleys and continue the trip slowly.

The rope would not function nearly as well as the original part, but would allow one to keep going. This is how toxic metals can function positively in the body, at times. Many people limp along on grossly deficient diets, and many today are born deficient in the vital minerals and too high in toxic metals due to imbalances in their mothers.

Their fatigue and other symptoms are due to the presence of incorrect "replacement parts" in their biological engine compartments. Depending on where toxic metals accumulate, the resulting effects may be given names such as hypothyroidism, diabetes or cancer. The idea of preferred minerals is discussed in a theoretical context in the article on this website entitled The Theory of Nutritional Balancing Science.

This is critical to understand. It means that toxic metals can have an adaptive function to sustain life in the face of vital mineral deficiencies. Nutritional balancing programs replace less preferred minerals with more preferred minerals. This therapy concept is not well-known.

3. Stress and toxic metals. Stress depletes vital minerals faster. This leads to deficiencies of these minerals. This, in turn, causes the body to absorb more toxic metals. In this way, stress is a direct cause of toxic metal excess, which in turn contributes or causes many health conditions, aging, disabilities and death.

4. Mineral antagonisms. Eating plenty of nutrient minerals actually antagonizes, or prevents the absorption of the toxic metals. Deficient diets, however, always result in toxic metal accumulation and poisoning because there are fewer vital minerals in refined food to compete with the toxic metals for absorption and utilization inside the body.

5. The anthropomorphic concept. All minerals, including the toxic metals, have very specific qualities that affect our bodies, and even our personalities, when we have a lot of the mineral inside us. For example, cadmium is a very hard toxic metal. Inside the body, it hardens the arteries and other tissues, and it even hardens a person's personality.

6. The poor eliminator concept. A key to solving toxic metal problem is to understand that many people cannot eliminate toxic metals very well. This fact is often overlooked when doctors try to correct toxic metal poisoning. The worst problem is not necessarily the presence of a toxic metal, but rather an inability to eliminate toxic metals. Hair mineral testing has very specific individual mineral indicators for poor ability to eliminate these metals.

7. Toxic forms of vital minerals. A confusing fact is that nutrient minerals such as chromium, manganese, iron, copper, potassium and even calcium and others can be in a form that is highly toxic to the body. In other words, nutrient minerals can be in a form that makes them act like toxic metals for the body. In most cases, the body cannot convert the toxic (oxide or other) form into a usable form. Instead, the body must eliminate the toxic forms of these minerals to restore health.

This can be very confusing for both practitioners and clients. For example, it may appear on a test as if one is eliminating a nutrient mineral. In reality, one is just eliminating a toxic form of a nutrient mineral that is damaging the body.

8. Developmental versus toxic minerals.
Toxic metals slow or stop what is called on this website development. This is a very special type of healing of the body. It is critical to replace the toxic metals with what we call the spiritual minerals such as zinc and selenium, in order to promote development. We call the latter spiritual minerals because they are needed for advanced brain activity. This topic is discussed in a separate article entitled Introduction to Development on this website.

Before discussing toxic metals, let us briefly discuss minerals, in general.

INTRODUCTION TO THE MINERALS

Minerals are the building blocks of our bodies. They are required for body structure, fluid balance, protein structures and to produce hormones. Minerals also act as co-factors, catalysts and inhibitors of all our body's enzymes. Everything in our bodies are made of about 50 minerals, also called chemical elements. Having the right minerals is a great a key to the health of every body system and function.

Mineral classification - Minerals are classified into four groups:

1. Macro-minerals. These are found in large quantity in our bodies. They include calcium, magnesium, sodium, potassium, phosphorus and sulfur. The first four are sometimes called the electrolytes, because they are common in the blood.

2. Required trace minerals - These include iron, copper, zinc, manganese, chromium, selenium, boron, silicon, iodine, vanadium, lithium, molybdenum, cobalt, germanium and perhaps a few others.

3. Possibly required trace minerals - Less is known about these. They may include rubidium, tin, niobium, gold, silver and others.

4. Toxic metals - The well-studied include aluminum, antimony, barium, beryllium, bismuth, bromine, cadmium, chlorine, fluoride, lead, mercury nickel, and uranium. However, there are a dozen or more others. However, a complete nutritional balancing program will remove many others such as germanium, gadolinium (used in MRI scans as a contrast medium), thallium, and others. This is a distinct advantage of this program over others that target only one or two toxic metals.

The categories of minerals above sometimes overlap slightly because assessing minerals that are required by humans is not a clear cut science. Some of them may be needed in minuscule amounts, for example. Also, some forms of the required minerals can be highly toxic. Examples are some forms of copper, iron, manganese, hexavalent chromium, se-

lenium and others. Too much of even the most needed minerals can also become toxic.

TOXIC METAL DANGERS

Easy exposure - Today mankind is exposed
to the highest levels in recorded history of lead, mercury, arsenic, aluminum, copper, nickel, tin, antimony, bromine, bismuth and vanadium, among others.
The levels are up to several thousand times higher
than in primitive man.

Persistent in the environment - Toxic metals
are also persistent. The late Henry Schroeder, MD,
who was a world authority on minerals, wrote:
"Most organic substances are degradable by
natural processes. (However), no metal is degradable…they are here to stay for a long time".

Persistent and cumulative in the body - Toxic
metals also tend to persist or remain in our bodies for
years. We can remove some of them if we are
healthy, but many also accumulate. This is the reason
why nutritional balancing program include what
some consider "drastic" measures to help eliminate
them such as coffee enemas, sauna therapy and certain supplements.

Specific types of damage:

Depositing in tissues - Toxic metals may also simply deposit in many sites, causing local irritation and other toxic effects.

Causing infection - Some toxic metals support development of fungal, bacterial and viral infections that are difficult or impossible to eradicate until this cause is removed.

Damaging biosynthesis - Toxic metals are very involved in the production of all chemicals in our bodies from DNA and RNA. They are needed as raw materials for body chemicals, for enzymes that participate in the synthesis of all of our chemicals, and for more. Toxic metals interfere, block, replace, and poison many aspects of biosynthesis.

Weakening body structures - For example, lead, fluoride, aluminum and other toxic metals that find their way into the bones weaken the bones.

General enzyme damage - Toxic metals replace nutrient minerals in enzyme binding sites. When this occurs, the metals inhibit, overstimulate or otherwise alter thousands of enzymes. An affected enzyme may operate at 5% of normal activity. This may contribute to many health conditions. Toxic metals may also replace other substances in other tissue structures. These tissues, such as the arteries, joints, bones and muscles, are weakened by the replacement process.

Other. Toxic metals upset digestion, alter gland activity, change the metabolic rate, and damage organs such as the kidneys and liver. In addition, all are neurotoxic. This means they damage the brain and nervous system. In fact, we find that many mental and emotional health disorders involve excess toxic metals in the body and brain. I hope that someday this fact will be recognized in the fields of psychology and psychiatry. There is a small group of doctors known as orthomolecular psychiatrists who are aware of this, but they are yet very few in number.

MODERN DIETS AND TOXIC METALS

The danger of toxic metals is greatly aggravated today by the low mineral content of most of our food supply. An abundance of vital minerals protects against toxic metals. Vital minerals compete with toxic metals for absorption and utilization in enzymes and other tissue structures.

However, when food is low in essential minerals, the body absorbs and makes use of more toxic metals. To continue the analogy from the previous section, we are not stocking up sufficiently on factory parts, so we must use the greatly inferior replacement parts – toxic metals. Causes for the low mineral content of almost all agricultural products are primarily:

1. Hybrid crops are bred for production or disease resistance, rather than superior nutrition.

2. Superphosphate fertilizers produce higher yields by stimulating growth, but the crops grown this way do not provide nearly as many trace elements. They are used on both commercial and organic crops. We do not replace all the trace minerals on our agricultural fields today. Instead, human and animal manures are often flushed into the rivers and oceans, where they do not belong and are often pollutants.

4. Toxic pesticides used on commercial farms damage soil microorganisms needed to help plants absorb minerals from the soil.

5. After harvesting crops, food refining and processing almost always reduce the mineral content of food. Whole wheat flour, when milled to make white flour, loses 40% of its chromium, 86% of its manganese, 89% of its cobalt, 78% of its zinc and 48% of its molybdenum.

Refining cane into sugar causes even greater losses. EDTA may be added to frozen foods to retain their color. However, this chelating agent removes minerals that otherwise would cause the surface minerals to 'tarnish', discoloring the vegetables.

As a result of the above, the term 'empty calories' aptly describes most of our food today, even some natural foods. Newer genetically-modified crops are even worse.

Please eat only whole, natural foods. Organically grown is almost always better. However, it can vary and many organic foods are still hybridized varieties.

SOURCES AND SYMPTOMS OF TOXIC METALS

ALUMINUM

Aluminum is called the soft in the head mineral because it is associated with memory loss and dementia. Aluminum is a very soft and dangerous toxic mineral. Aluminum is everywhere, and almost everyone shows some aluminum toxicity on hair tests. Among the most important sources are all types of salt. Table salt also often has aluminum added as an anti-caking agent and should never be eaten!

Sea salt is better - I like one called Real Salt by Redmond, which has less aluminum than some others. Cities routinely add aluminum to their tap water as a flocculating agent (to remove dirt particles). This is a horrible practice. Modern anti-perspirants all contain toxic aluminum compounds. The deodorant stones and deodorant crystals are no better, even though they are "natural". Use an old-fashioned deodorant instead, or spray some dilute hydrogen peroxide or some liquid soap like Dr. Bronner's soap under your arms instead.

Beverages in aluminum cans or food cooked in aluminum may contain elevated levels of aluminum. Aluminum is also used in some baking powders, and other products. Peppermint, spearmint and wintergreen teas are rather high in aluminum. For much more detail about aluminum, read Aluminum and Aluminum, Iron and Manganese – The Amigos on this website.

ARSENIC

I call arsenic the slow death mineral. Its symptoms are vague, and it was used to kill people because it is colorless and tasteless, so it was added to food and slowly killed people. Today, arsenic is still a common toxin. It may legally be added to chicken feed (Roxsarone) according to the corrupt US Food and Drug Administration (the FDA) and the somewhat corrupt US Department of Agriculture (USDA). I believe Europe has banned arsenic in chicken feed.

Arsenic can get into commercial eggs, all pig products such as pork, ham, bacon and lard, and into most US drinking water supplies as it leaches into the soil from farming and livestock operations. Organic chicken and eggs should be better. Avoid all pig products due to parasite problems, even if well-cooked, and to avoid the arsenic.

Arsenic is used in pesticides and, as a result, may be found in commercial wines, beers, fruits, vegetables, rice and other foods. Once again, organically grown should be better. Recently, rice grown in China has been found to be quite contaminated with arsenic. For much more on this topic read Arsenic Toxicity and the USDA/FDA Cover-up and Arsenic on this website.

BROMINE

Among the many food sources of bromine are breads and clear-colored soda pop. These include Mountain Dew, Crystal Light, Sprite and others. Bromine can damage the thyroid gland and replace iodine in all body tissues. This is quite serious. It should not be allowed to be added to our foods. Read Bromine for more details.

CADMIUM

We call cadmium the macho mineral, and it is one of the violent elements. Cadmium toughens the tissues and hardens the arteries. It also hardens the personality. Like lead, it is an older male mineral that is associated with macho behavior, violence and horror. The concept that when we ingest or are exposed to a toxic metal, our bodies and our minds take on the qualities of the mineral is called the anthropomorphic quality of minerals. It means that each mineral – both the vital minerals and the toxic metals – have human-like qualities such as hardness, softness, or malleability, and they influence us.

Interestingly, cadmium helps people to "be tough" and take risks. For example, many modern city women have high cadmium that allows them to function in male-oriented jobs such as being company executives. Cadmium helps them and others, such as prostitutes, to act more tough and to handle lots of stress.

Military men and women, and police often have more cadmium, as it helps them handle their very difficult jobs, at times, and take risks. Unfortunately, it is also a deadly toxic metal associated with heart disease, cancers of all kind, kidney disease, diabetes and other serious health problems.

People who have orgasms more than once a week tend to accumulate more cadmium, probably because cadmium replaces zinc in the male testicles, and even in women's ovaries. Male and female sexual fluids are rich in zinc and some cadmium.

Cadmium is widespread in the air, as it is used in brake linings of cars. It is also used in metal plating as it is a very hard substance. Tobacco cigarette, marijuana and CBD oil or cannabis oil contain cadmium. This is one reason people like marijuana, as cadmium boosts the sodium level. They don't realize they are poisoning themselves – usually permanently – by using it. Cadmium is also used as a catalyst in some hydrogenated products such as commercial peanut butter and margarine. Please avoid these horrible food items. For much more about cadmium read Cadmium on this website.

LEAD

Lead is called the horror mineral because it is associated with violence, lowered IQ, attention deficit disorder, hyperactivity, and many other neurological problems. Lead is a widely distributed toxic metal due to its many uses in industry.

Pesticides used on fruits, vegetables and many other foods may contain lead, among other toxic metals. Lead was added to gasoline until the 1970s in the USA and elsewhere. Now gasoline contains a highly toxic form of manganese, instead.

Old house paint, current paint used on ships of all sizes, a few hair dyes, lubricants, medications, cosmetics such as lipstick and others, inks, and perhaps other products may contain lead. Glazes used on cookware in some nations still contain lead that can come off onto the food.

MERCURY

Mercury may be called the mad hatters mineral. People who made raccoon skin hats in the mid-1800s in America and Europe developed mercury toxicity after a few years from rubbing mercury on felt to soften it. They became mentally and emotionally deranged, in many cases.

"Silver" dental amalgam fillings are usually about half mercury. I would have them replaced if you have them, as the mercury will slowly leach out of them and into your body.

Fish and seafood is universally contaminated with mercury. It is really a tragedy, since otherwise it is a great food. Mercury is found today in ALL FISH, bar none. Even small fish, which used to be safe, are not any more.

As a result, the only fish I suggest eating are sardines. For details of why, read Sardines on this site. I suggest avoiding all other fish. I know there is a problem because anyone who eats fish other than these on a regular basis, even once a week, demonstrates high mercury on a hair mineral test. Indeed, large fish concentrate mercury a million times or more. The federal government recently issued a warning that pregnant and lactating women should avoid tuna, shark, king mackerel, halibut, ahi, Mahi Mahi, and other large fish. Avoid shellfish. Shellfish are often even more toxic than other fish. For some reason, their bodies often accumulate cadmium and lead, in addition to mercury. Most shellfish are caught in coastal waters, which are the most contaminated. Please avoid all shellfish, forever, as the problem is just getting worse in most nations of the world.

Once again, this is sad to have to say, but mineral tests reveal the problem to anyone willing to check my assertion. This is why many people are "allergic" to them. This is a mild term. They are really poisoned by them. For much more detail about mercury, read Mercury on this website.

NICKEL

This is called the depression and suicide mineral, as it is associated with these feelings and symptoms. Nickel is another hardener, used to plate inexpensive jewelry, in coins, and as a plating material for bathroom fixtures and many other metallic items. Most orthodontic braces sadly contain nickel today. It is also found in some metal crowns and dental wires used in bridges and elsewhere in dentistry. Be very careful about this because nickel can contribute to cancer and other health problems.

Nickel is found in rooibos tea or red tea. It is also used as a catalyst to make ALL hydrogenated oil products such as commercial peanut butter, ALL margarines, and vegetable shortening. For much more detail about nickel, read Nickel on this website.

FLUORIDE

Fluoride is sometimes called a cancer mineral. It is highly toxic. In fact, it is sold as rat poison. The research about its toxicity and horror for the human body is very clear scientifically, but this is suppressed by most public health authorities in the USA and Great Britain. The biggest source is fluoride added to drinking water supplies. Adding fluoride to drinking water not only does not stop cavities in the teeth. It is totally insane, because fluoride compounds added to drinking water are extremely toxic.

Most of the world has stopped this awful practice except for parts of America and Great Britain. More and more Western cities and towns are voting it out. If your town still has it, organize to get rid of it. Several excellent websites and organizations are there to help.

Fluorides have found their way into ground water supplies, and thus into the food chain. For this reason, fluoride levels in foods processed with water may be very high, especially baby foods and reconstituted vegetable and fruit juices. Please never consume these, and never feed them to your children. Also, do not give babies and children fluoride tablets or fluoride treatments at the dentist's office.

Health authorities, who recommend fluoridating the water, or any fluorides, are extremely ignorant, in my experience. I have debated dentists and public health officials on this issue. Their real level of knowledge of the medical literature on fluorides is lacking.

Recommendation for fluoride also rarely, if ever, take into account the already toxic amount of fluorides people are already getting in natural foods, foods processed with fluoridated water, and fluoridated toothpaste and mouthwashes. The combination adds up to overload, in all cases.

Hydrofluosilicic acid, the chemical often used to fluoridate drinking water, is a smokestack waste that contains lead, mercury, cadmium, arsenic, aluminum, benzene and radioactive waste material. For much more on this horror please read Fluoridation of the Water on this site.

CHLORINE

Everyone assumes chlorine is safe, since it is used to purify most all drinking water around the world. It is not safe, however. It is a very toxic mineral associated with heart disease and dementia, among other health conditions. Purification of water supplies with ozone is much better. I strongly suggest that everyone drink either spring water, which has little to no chlorine in it, or drink carbon-only filtered tap or other water.

Carbon will remove most chlorine from water. A carbon block filter is best. Just remember to change the filter every few months so it will keep working. Note that carbon and carbon block filters do not remove most toxic metals from water. Only distillation and reverse osmosis remove most toxic metals. However, these produce mineral-free water that is not good to drink for this reason, and for other reasons, as well.

Another important source of toxic chlorine is the residue found in bleached flour and any products such as bread, pastry, cookies and more made with bleached white flour. Chlorine is used to bleach the flour.

COPPER

Copper is not a toxic metal. However, it often accumulates in toxic forms in the body, and causes many health problems. This problem is extremely common today. Copper mainly accumulates in the nervous system and in the female organs. For example, copper toxicity is associated with migraine headaches, premenstrual syndrome, depression, anxiety, panic attacks, some schizophrenias and seizures.

Copper also can replace selenium in various tissues. This can impair the conversion of T4 to T3, contributing to thyroid imbalances that are very common. For much more about copper please read Copper Toxicity Syndrome on this website.

IRON

Iron is a vital mineral. However, acquired iron toxicity is extremely common. This is what we find on hair mineral tests. This is not the same as the genetic disease hemochromatosis. The toxicity has a different cause. The iron is in a toxic form, often in an oxide form that is very irritating and pro-inflammatory. Sources include eating red meat more than about twice or three times weekly or eating more than 4-5 ounce portions of it. Other sources are taking iron pills or mineral supplements containing iron.

Another important source is "iron-enriched" foods such as breads and most other products made with white flour. Some herbs such as black cohosh are high in iron, as is some drinking water. Iron can give drinking water a slight yellowish color. Holding on to anger can increase iron in the body. Many babies today are born with too much toxic iron, just as they are born with too much of many toxic substances.

Holistic doctors often give anti-oxidants to help reduce the inflammation. However, a much better solution is to remove the toxic iron. Nutritional balancing programs do this, in all cases. However, other nutritional, herbal or medical programs cannot do this very well, in my experience.

URANIUM

The main sources of uranium are air polluted with radioactive particles from A-bomb tests, nuclear power plant emissions, nuclear plant accidents such as the Fukishima disaster recently in Japan, and perhaps some foods contaminated with uranium from the same sources. Uranium is radioactive, as is radon gas found in some homes. It can damage the lungs and other organs; it damages DNA, and is associated with higher levels of cancer and other diseases.

General Food Sources. Food grown near highways or downwind of industrial plants may contain lead and other toxic amounts of metals. Even organic home gardens may be contaminated if, for example, old house paint containing lead leaches lead into the soil.

Sprays and insecticides still often contain lead, arsenic, mercury and other toxic metals. Refining of food often contaminates the food with aluminum, as it is found in water supplies everywhere and it may be used in some food refining processes. Also, some food refining removes the protective zinc, chromium and manganese from food and leaves the toxic metals in some cases, such as cadmium. This makes white flour even more toxic, as with white sugar, and is another reason to totally avoid these foods.

Airborne Sources of Toxic Metals - Most toxic metals are effectively absorbed by inhalation. Auto, ship and aircraft exhaust, industrial smoke and products from incinerators are among the airborne sources of toxic metals and other chemicals. Mercury and coal-fired power plants - Burning coal can release mercury, lead and cadmium among other metals. Iranian and Venezuelan oil are high in vanadium. Coal plants should have scrubbers, as they do in the United States. However, India and China, in particular, often do not have scrubbers on their power plants. They may not realize the damage their plants are causing to the entire world due to pollution of the air, water and food supplies.

Uranium exposure is largely from airborne sources such as nuclear bomb tests and accidents at nuclear power plants. All nuclear power plants also emit some low-level radiation from uranium refining and medical use of nuclear material. X-rays, CT scans, PET scans and dental x-rays also add to our burden of ionizing radiation today. Fortunately, some of this can be removed with a nutritional balancing program.

Incineration can be clean - Older methods of incineration of electronic parts, plastics, treated fabrics, batteries and even diapers release all the toxic metals into the air. The use of scrubbers and newer methods of very high temperature incineration are much better. Cadmium and mercury in papers - Cigarette and marijuana smoke are high in cadmium, and cadmium is found in cigarette and joint rolling paper. It helps keep the drugs burning. Pesticides used on these crops may contain lead, arsenic and other toxic metals.

Medications and toxic metals - Many prescription and over-the-counter drugs contain toxic metals. Cipro (fluoquinolone antibiotics) and antidepressants such as Prozac (fluoxetine) are fluoride-containing drugs, for example. Thimerosal, a mercury-containing preservative, is still used in many vaccines, including most flu shots, even when doctors deny it, I am told. Independent evaluation of a large study that is part of the Centers for Disease Control Vaccine Safety Datalink concluded that:

"Children are 27 times as likely to develop autism after exposure to three thimerisol-containing vaccines than those who receive thimerisol-free versions".

Thiazide diuretics contain mercury. These include Maxzide, Diazide and many others. Antacids such as Ryopan, Gaviscon, Maalox, Mylanta and many others are very high in aluminum. Direct Skin Contact As A Source Of Toxic Metals. Almost all anti-perspirants and many cosmetics contain aluminum. Dental amalgams contain mercury, copper and other metals. Dental bridges and other appliances often contain nickel. Prostheses and pins used to hold bones together may contain nickel and other toxic metals, although most are titanium and stainless steel, which are much better.

Copper intra-uterine devices (IUDs) release lots of copper into the body. This can cause depression and other problems for some women. Soaps, body lotions and creams often contain toxic compounds. A few hair dyes and commercial high-end lipsticks contain lead. Selsun Blue shampoo contains selenium that is quite toxic. Head N Shoulders shampoo is much safer and contains zinc, but not selenium. Household lawn and garden chemicals may contain lead, arsenic and other compounds. Mercury treated seeds and arsenic-treated wood are other common sources of toxic metals.

Occupational exposure to toxic metals is important for many occupations today. Among the worst are plumbers, electricians, auto mechanics, printers, ironworkers, and other metal workers. Workers need to wear gloves, masks and take other precautions when handling inks, metals and other toxic materials.

CONGENITAL TOXIC METALS

This is an extremely important and preventable tragedy. Today, all children are born with some toxic metals acquired in utero. All the toxic metals pass through the placenta from mother to child. This is seen clearly when reviewing mineral analyses of infants. These are babies who have never been exposed to food, yet their bodies are high in many toxic metals.

The only explanation is that these infants receive exposures in utero during gestation. This is a very sad situation, as many children are born with two strikes against them, so to speak. They are far more prone to autism, ADD, ADHD, infections, developmental delays and more.

This tragedy can be largely prevented if all young women would go on a nutritional balancing program combined with yoga/meditation practices before they become pregnant to reduce their load of toxic metals. It does not matter how healthy a woman appears to be. Most all young women today have too many toxic metals in the body that are passed on to their children. The problem of congenital toxic metals is especially important because standard prenatal care is horribly lacking in Western nations

DETECTING TOXIC METALS

Toxic metals are not easy to detect. In fact, detecting all the toxic metals is impossible, because they accumulate deep within body tissues and organs. Here are comments on the various methods of detection, including tests of the blood, urine, hair, feces, liver biopsy tests, and other methods such as electrical machines and applied kinesiology.

Blood tests - The problem with blood tests is that the body quickly removes toxic metals from the blood and moves them into the tissues. So blood tests must be done soon after an exposure, usually within days or weeks at the most, or they are practically useless. Blood tests are helpful for an acute exposure, such as eating a food contaminated with lead and doing a test soon after. However, this entire article is mainly about chronic toxic metal poisoning.

Urine and feces challenge tests. These are done by first administering a chelation drug that binds to and removes toxic metals. Examples are EDTA or DMPS, for example. Then one collects a 24-hour urine, or a feces sample to see what comes out of the body. This test does not detect most toxic metals. The reason is that the chelating drugs mainly circulate in the blood. So they tend to miss most toxic metals that are stored in the tissues or incorporated into enzymes in the brain, heart, liver, kidneys and elsewhere.

Liver or other biopsies - This method is more accurate and is used, at times, to detect iron poisoning and copper poisoning, for example. However, liver biopsies are costly, invasive and somewhat dangerous. For this reason, liver biopsies are not used often. Electrical machines - Electroacupuncture devices, radionics machines and other machines can detect some toxic metals.

Applied kinesiology - This method, also called muscle testing, is variable in its reliability and extremely dependent upon the operator or practitioner. It also does not quantify the amount of metals present. I would not depend upon it.

HAIR MINERAL ANALYSIS FOR TOXIC METAL DETECTION

The hair test measures toxic metals deposited in the hair and skin. Fortunately, if a person follow a complete nutritional balancing program, all the toxic metals come out of the body, so figuring out which are present is not too important.

Why hair? Hair accumulates toxic metals because hair is an excretory tissue. This means that anything that goes into the hair will be removed from the body. So the body often unloads poisons by shunting them into the hair and skin.

The hair mineral test is also unique in that it is a biopsy type of test that gives a snapshot of the inside of the body cells. None of the other methods do this so directly.

Government opinion on hair testing. The United States Environmental Protection Agency or EPA reviewed over 400 studies of the use of hair for toxic metal detection and concluded that:

"Hair is a meaningful and representative tissue for (biological monitoring for) antimony, arsenic, cadmium, chromium, copper, lead, mercury, nickel, vanadium and perhaps selenium and tin. "

The author of a study of lead toxicity in Massachusetts school children, Dr. R. Tuthill, concluded:

"Scalp hair should be considered a useful clinical and epidemiological approach for the measurement of chronic low-level lead exposure in children."

Reading the levels of the toxic metals on a hair analysis report is not sufficient to glean all the information from the test. Here is how to do it better:

1. The hair must be washed at home within 48 hours or less before sampling. Any ordinary shampoo may be used. If one has a water softener, then it is best to wash the hair twice before sampling it, using unsoften tap water, reverse osmosis water, distilled or spring water.

2. The hair sample must not be washed at the laboratory at all. The reason is that washing the hair always erratically removes some of its minerals.

3. Look for elevated levels of toxic metals. However,

MOST LABORATORIES HAVE THEIR AC-CEPTABLE LEVELS OF TOXIC METALS SET TOO HIGH. One must use the acceptable levels that are listed in the section below.

4. The amigos. These are toxic forms of iron, manganese and aluminum. The interpretation rule is that if any one of these is elevated, the other two are elevated in the body as well. Elevated aluminum is any reading above 0.04 mg% or 0.4 ppm. Elevated iron is any reading above 2 mg% or 20 ppm. Elevated manganese is any reading above 0.04 mg% or 0.4 ppm. Read more about this interesting situation in The Amigos or Oxidants– Iron, Manganese and Aluminum.

5. Poor eliminator patterns. An excellent indicator of hidden toxic metals in the body is the presence of a poor eliminator pattern. For the exact criteria for these patterns, read Poor Eliminator Pattern.

6. Hidden copper toxicity. The hair copper level is a very poor indicator of copper toxicity. Instead, look for hidden copper indicators, which include:

- Copper greater than 2.5 mg% or 25 ppm.
- Copper less than 1.5 mg% or 15 ppm.
- Calcium greater than about 65 mg% or 650 ppm.

- Potassium less than about 5 mg% or 50 ppm.
- Mercury greater than about 0.035 mg% or 0.35 ppm.
- Zinc less than 13 mg% or 130 ppm.
- Na/K ratio less than 2.0
- Four lows pattern.
- Zinc greater than 17 mg% or 170 ppm, in many cases.
- Phosphorus less than 12 mg% or 120 ppm, in most cases.

7. Mercury indicators. Mercury is so widespread that almost everyone has too much. I do not pay too much attention to any test for mercury because I know that:

a) Anyone who eats large or medium-sized fish has a lot.

b) Anyone with amalgam dental fillings has a lot.

c) Anyone who eats seafood or sushi has plenty.

d) Most, if not all babies today are born with it thanks to toxicity in their mothers.

The hair or other test results are often not as important as these dietary, lifestyle and environmental factors.

8. Other general indicators of high toxic metals on a hair mineral analysis. These include a very slow oxidation rate, fast oxidation in an adult, three highs or four highs pattern, and sympathetic dominance pattern.

I realize this includes almost everyone, and that is the truth. We know this because even those who show few toxic metals on their initial hair mineral test often eliminate large quantities of toxic metals during nutritional balancing programs. This shows itself on repeat hair mineral tests, and often takes a number of years to be revealed.

In one of the case studies, it took eight years before cadmium showed up on patient's hair test, and about 20 years before nickel showed up.

HIGH, LOW AND NORMAL HAIR LEVELS FOR THE TOXIC METALS

AGING AND TOXIC METALS

The slow, or not so slow, replacement of vital minerals with toxic metals is an important and neglected cause of aging due to deactivation of enzyme systems and the loss of organ and tissue integrity. One could say it is the essence of aging, from a purely mineral perspective.

Toxic metal accumulation also feeds on itself. As one's energy production decreases with age, the body is less able to eliminate toxic metals. This, in turn, causes more metal accumulation.

GENETICS, GENE EXPRESSION AND TOXIC METALS

Many birth defects are due to faulty gene expression and not DNA problems. Toxic metals are one cause. For example, zinc is required for several key enzymes in gene expression, such as RNA transferee and RNA polymerase. Not surprisingly, zinc deficiency is associated with conditions such as neural tube defects. Many toxic metals interfere with zinc metabolism.

Single nucleotide polymorphisms or SNPs are a fancy name for defective gene expression, even though the DNA is fine. Toxic metals at the cellular level can cause these.

SOLUTIONS TO TOXIC METAL OVER-LOAD

One should not fear toxic metals. They cannot be completely avoided, but one can minimize exposure with careful eating and a healthful lifestyle. Also, our bodies have a lot of evolutionary experience with them and effective mechanisms to eliminate them. These can be supported and enhanced with a nutritional balancing program. This method, which does not involve chelation at all, uses at least 35 methods together, at once, to remove ALL toxic metals safely and deeply. In my experience, it is more thorough, safer and removes metals better than intravenous or any other type of chelation therapy. Also, all chelating agents remove some beneficial minerals along with the toxic ones. For more on why I do not like chelation therapy, read Chelation Therapy.

HOW TO DETOXIFY THE BODY

The methods below are always used together in nutritional balancing program, in an integrated combination, to remove all toxic metals and hundreds of toxic chemicals, as well, from the body.

1. Increase the amount of rest and sleep greatly. Extra rest and sleep is critical for any detoxification program for several reasons:

a) Detoxification takes place mostly when we are resting or sleeping. During the day when one is active, the body is mainly focused on the daily activities, not on eliminating poisons from the body.

b) Rest and sleep reduce sympathetic nervous system activity. This is so important it is listed separately as a powerful method to enhance detoxification of all chemicals, metals and other types of poisons.

c) Resting and sleeping more conserves the body's energy for healing. Most people use up too much energy in their daily activities. This slows progress tremendously.

d) The essential organs and glands, such as the adrenals, thyroid, liver, kidneys and others rebuild best when rested.

e) Sleep allows mental and emotional processing to occur. This reduces stress, which helps release toxic metals. Many people live in continual stress because they do not process each day's events and traumas enough at night due to not enough resting time.

2. Inhibit the sympathetic nervous system. This is another key to our programs. Sympathetic nervous system activity reduces the elimination of all toxins from the body. This is well known in medicine.

The liver, kidneys, bowel, and skin even the lungs are all associated with the parasympathetic nervous system. They are also important organs of elimination. Sympathetic nervous system activity inhibits these activities powerfully. One can reduce sympathetic activity in at least six ways:

a) As mentioned above, get a lot more rest and sleep. This is a primary method of reducing sympathetic nervous system activity.

b) Diet is important needs to be as nourishing and non-stimulatory as possible. Lots of cooked vegetables provide the most minerals possible.

The diet also needs to minimize chemical additives and other toxins. One should also limit caffeine, sugar, wheat, most beef, and other stimulating, irritating, allergic or sensitive foods in the diet.

c) Supplements used in nutritional balancing programs are carefully chosen to have a parasympathetic effect. This means strictly limiting all stimulating products, including many herbs, as well.

d) The lifestyle must be restful in general. This can have a big influence on the nervous system, even if one sleeps enough. It includes one's activities, relationships, job or career, thoughts and emotions.

e) Practicing Yoga regularly is very helpful to reduce sympathetic nervous system activity. Regular prayer, certain affirmations, and always watching one's "mental diet" can be critical to reduce fear, anger and negativity. Too much that is on the television, the news and other information sources are harmful to the body's delicate nervous system.

f) Other ways to reduce sympathetic nervous stimulation are to be careful with excessive exercise, reduce cell phone use, and avoid other radiation sources. Far infrared saunas give off harmful EM fields and should not be used.

Red heat lamp saunas, however, are excellent to reduce sympathetic nervous system activity. Reduce noise levels, freeway driving and other more dangerous or unnerving activities. These and many other simple changes together can reduce your stress level dramatically.

g) Reducing certain imbalances on a hair mineral chart also can dramatically lower sympathetic nervous activity. These include, but are not limited to, balancing a fast oxidation rate, reducing a high Na/K or a high Ca/Mg ratio, improving zinc, selenium and chromium status and lowering certain toxic metal levels.

3. Eat an excellent-quality diet of 70-80% cooked vegetables and some animal protein daily. Avoid all fruits, fruit juices, sweets, most nuts and seeds and strictly avoid vegetarian and raw food diets.

This diet is the richest in alkaline reserve minerals that I know of. The body will absorb and utilize less toxic metals if it receives more of the preferred minerals. A recent study in the Journal of Clinical Nutrition measured the mineral content of organic versus commercial food. Results indicated that food labeled "organic" that was selected randomly from Chicago food markets had an average of twice the mineral content of standard supermarket food.

The famed people of Hunza who live to 120 years or longer in excellent health drink glacial runoff that was so mineral-rich the water was cloudy (see The Wheel of Health by G.T. Wrench, paperback edition, 2009). Other mineral-rich foods that are part of the diets we recommend are kelp, sea salt, and bone broth. The fiber from cooked vegetables and whole grains reduces bowel transit time and reduces constipation, which help limit the absorption of toxic metals.

4. Other dietary considerations. These include;

a) Avoid all restrictive and extreme diets. These include strict vegan and vegetarian diets, for example. Raw food diets do not work well today because no one is able to extract enough minerals from raw foods. The minerals are not available because they are bound up with tough vegetable fibers that we cannot properly digest, even with a digestive aid.

Cooking does not reduce the mineral content of food and usually makes minerals much more bioavailable by breaking down fiber. Cooking also con-

centrates the food so that one ends up ingesting
many more vital minerals.

b) Avoid living on protein powders and other processed supplements instead of foods. For example, egg or whey protein powder is not a substitute for eating eggs or fresh goat milk. The latter are
whole foods that are much richer in many minerals.
Food supplements are never a substitute for an excellent diet.

c) Avoid most refined foods such as white
sugar, white flour, table salt and white rice. These
are almost devoid of vital minerals and will cause the
body to absorb and utilize more toxic metals.

5. Improve the eating habits, attitudes and
other aspects of lifestyle. Excellent eating habits include having regular, sit-down meals in a quiet place.
Also, eat quietly and slowly, and chew thoroughly.
These habits assist nutrient absorption and proper
elimination. Poor habits include skipping meals,
snacking all day, eating on the run, and eating the
same foods every day with no variety.

Attitudes - A relaxed and positive outlook
greatly facilitates elimination and healing of all illness. One's attitudes can matter greatly as well.
They either relieve stress, or add to it. I encourage an
attitude of gratitude and avoidance of all victims
thinking. This includes thinking that anyone else is a
victim, either. Such apparently small changes in
one's thoughts and actions can have a huge impact

on general health and the body's ability to heal and eliminate toxic substances. In contrast, hopelessness and low self-esteem impair elimination. These factors are too often overlooked by medical and holistic practitioners. In some cases, other lifestyle patterns are destructive and must be changed, such as drinking too much alcohol, recreational drug use, spending time with negative or destructive "friends", and other lifestyle issues.

6. Nutritional supplements - Nutritional supplements called mineral antagonists can help reduce toxic metals in the body. For example, kelp is an inexpensive source of iodine that can help remove fluorides, chlorides and bromides from the body by competing with them for absorption and for binding sites in the cells of the body.

Kelp also contains alginates that help bind toxic metals in the intestines so they will be removed. Kelp also contains a wide range of other vital minerals to body needs to rebuild it. All act as antagonists to some degree to the toxic metals.

In addition to kelp, nutritional balancing programs usually involve supplemental zinc, selenium, calcium, magnesium and other minerals. Calcium and zinc are cadmium antagonists. Selenium and zinc are mercury antagonists, and so on.

In nutritional balancing science, however, supplements must only be used in a way that does not unbalance the oxidation rate and the major mineral ratios. This is a major difference between this method and most other nutritional methods of healing.

The reason for this is that unbalancing the major mineral ratios decreases a person's vitality, which will negate or at least reduce the effectiveness of the entire program. Also, one must be careful not to use too many supplements. This adds too much yin energy to the body and can confuse the body. Also, many supplements subtly negate each other. For example, copper and vitamin C are definite antagonists. Therefore, supplementation must be kept simple and clearly follow these and other rules.

7. Support the eliminative organs. This greatly facilitates toxic metal removal. Balancing the mineral levels and ratios on a hair analysis is a powerful support for the eliminative organs. In addition, for the liver and bowel, we always give ox bile and pancreatic. We sometimes use a kidney support formula to support elimination through the kidneys.

The procedures such as red heat lamp sauna therapy, coffee enemas, foot reflexology and the Surya Namashkar Exercise also support the eliminative organs.

8. General nutritional support. In addition to the above, nutritional balancing programs always include general nutritional support such as vitamin D, omega-3 fatty acids and other nutrients. Food alone does not provide enough of these to replenish our demineralized bodies.

9. Improve adaptive energy. Increasing the amount of energy available to the body cells is a great key to toxic metal and toxic chemical elimination. The body must produce plenty of biochemical energy in order to eliminate toxins. This is sometimes overlooked by physicians, even holistic ones.

10. Balance the oxidation rate. The primary way to enhance adaptive energy using nutritional balancing science involves a properly performed and properly interpreted hair mineral analysis. With it, one can identify the oxidation type and the oxidation rate. One can then use foods, lifestyle, diet and other methods to balance the oxidation rate. This gentle balancing procedure, done in all nutritional balancing programs, greatly enhances the body's ability to eliminate toxic metals. For more on this topic, read Fast, Slow and Mixed Oxidation.

One must also avoid any supplement or procedure to remove toxins that upsets the oxidation rate. I teach this science to anyone who is interested. Click on the link, Training, for more information about learning this method.

11. Reduce exposure to toxic substances as much as possible. This includes exposures in foods, such as pesticide residues on foods, and chemical additives in foods. It includes pure water, if possible. However, I differ from some health authorities on this issue. The only water I recommend is either spring water or carbon-only filtered tap water. This includes soaps, lotions, cosmetics, creams and all skin

products. It also includes dental amalgam removal, except in the case of active cancer, which can be made worse by amalgam removal. Wait until the cancer is under control before doing this and preferably be on a nutritional balancing program to help reduce the side effects of amalgam removal. Some people also need to reduce occupational exposure to toxic metals.

12. Improve circulation, oxygenation and hydration. This is done with sauna therapy, deep breathing, the correct type and amount of drinking water, mild exercise (more is not needed and just wastes energy), and improving general health. Also, inhibiting the sympathetic nervous system assists with circulation.

13. Balancing yin and yang qualities in the body, and in one's life, in general. The concept of balance between opposite forces is one of the most ancient teachings on planet earth. It is critical for detoxification of heavy metals.

14. Distilled water, on occasion, but only during healing crises or purification reactions. Drinking distilled water will remove some loosely bound toxic metals. However, it can deplete essential minerals in the body because it is mineral-free water. Therefore, it is recommended during a healing reaction and when a person is already following a nutritional balancing program. At these times, it can be used for a few days or perhaps a week to reduce elimination

symptoms and speed up the removal of certain toxins from the body.

15. Remove the need for compensations and adaptations. This is a little more technical. Often, toxic metals perform an adaptive role in the body. They can support the activity of the adrenal glands, for example, and they can actually be used in some of the body's millions of enzyme systems to a limited extent.

By balancing the body chemistry delicately, the need for a toxic metal in an adaptive role can be removed. This makes possible the removal of many toxic metals. This methodology is built into nutritional balancing programs that are correctly designed.

16. Reduce all stress. Stress of any kind will slow the removal toxic metals. Therefore, reducing all stress on the body and mind greatly enhances toxin elimination.

17. Replace less preferred minerals with more preferred minerals. This is also a somewhat more complex topic. For each metallic-enzyme in the body, there are one or perhaps two preferred metals or minerals that will cause the enzyme to function optimally. Nutritional balancing programs always seek to replace less preferred minerals in enzyme binding sites with more preferred minerals. This is required for all deep healing. It is done by giving the appropriate foods and supplementary nutrients, avoiding the others, reducing toxic exposures and

stress, conserving energy for healing with more rest, and other methods.

18. Increase the body temperature when it is low. This may not seem important, but it is a very powerful method of enhancing many body activities, including elimination. Indeed, all the body's enzyme systems function optimally when the body temperature is ideal. However, most people have a low body temperature today, due in part to toxic metal accumulation in the thyroid and adrenal glands. Other reasons are fatigue, a low thyroid for other reason, nutrient depletion and others.

One can use a sauna to heat the body a few degrees every day. Even if it is only for 30-60 minutes at a time, this can have a tremendous effect of normalizing enzymatic reactions in the body that, in turn, promote healing and detoxification.

19. Eliminate infections and parasites of all kinds. This may not seem related to toxic metal removal, but it is. Most people have several dozen chronic infections in their bodies. Common sites are the eyes, ears, throat, bronchioles, intestines, teeth, and bladder. Each of these infections uses up adaptive energy or vitality in the body. As they are cleared using nutritional balancing – and never antibiotics that tend to be toxic – a person's vitality increases and his ability to then eliminate toxic metals increases, at times drastically.

20. Emotional and mental cleansing. This is an unusual concept, but can be vital to detoxify the body. We find that cadmium, for example, is associated with what may be called 'macho' styles of thinking. If a person will do the pushing down exercise, or just read the Bible, for example, it will help to release negative and violent thoughts. This will help remove some cadmium from the body. Similarly, copper toxicity is associated with fearful thoughts. If one reduces fearful thinking, then this will help reduce copper overload in the body.

21. Bridging over damaged enzymes. This is a very important mechanism whereby by giving higher doses of some vitamins, especially B-complex vitamins, one can bridge across enzymes damaged by the presence of toxic metals. These enzymes are needed to help remove the toxic metals.

22. The use of a powerful digestive aid for everyone. No matter how good the food one eats, if digestion is weak, and it is weak in almost everyone today, one will not absorb enough minerals and other nutrients. Insisting on a powerful digestive aid is therefore essential for many people to facilitate proper mineral absorption.

23. Integrating all of the above methods in a way so that none interferes with the others. This is essential. A problem with many medical and holistic approaches to toxic metal removal is that the methods of detoxification get in each other's way, which negates some or even all of the benefit. For example,

chelation is effective to remove some metals. However, most chelation, even natural chelating agents, removes some vital minerals along with the toxic ones. This is extremely harmful, and it is not an easy problem to solve. Simply taking minerals does not seem to work adequately. One reason is that minerals are complex, are found in many forms, and are best absorbed from food, not formulated products, in general.

Another problem with chelation is that the chelators are often slightly toxic, which damages the kidneys, liver and other organs, interfering with metal elimination. Chelation may also mobilize toxins from relatively harmless areas of the body and redistribute some in the kidneys, and this is harmful, as well.

24. Release traumas. This is most helpful for detoxification. It is a large subject, but the main idea is that when traumas are present, they directly interfere with elimination in the body because they affect the nervous system. Nutritional balancing releases most traumas fairly easily. For details, read Trauma Release on this site.

25. Release toxins in the body's own sequence, order and its own timing. This is extremely helpful to make the process of toxic metal removal as safe as possible, and more effective, as well. It is accomplished in nutritional balancing programs by focusing on raising the body's energy and vitality level, rather than focusing on pushing out particular

toxic metals. As the body's adaptive energy level rises, the body decides which metals to remove first.

26. Correct latent diseases and disorders. Nutritional balancing causes the healing of latent or sub-clinical health problems. This is an unusual ability of this program and depends upon raising the adaptive energy level of the body. Once these heal, the body is more capable of thorough detoxification. For example, many people have slightly damaged livers or slightly damaged kidneys. Yet the damage is sub-clinical or latent, meaning it does not cause any symptoms. When a person begins a nutritional balancing program, often these sub-clinical conditions are corrected first because they are the basis for later healing.

27. Other natural and balancing therapies. Therapies that combine beautifully with nutritional balancing include gentle chiropractic, osteopathic manipulation, Rolfing, structural integration, and foot and hand reflexology. These can help to reduce stress, improve vitality, support the eliminative organs, improves circulation and more.

RESTORING THE LIVER, KIDNEYS, SKIN AND LARGE INTESTINE

Many toxic metals accumulate in these organs. In most Westerns, in particular, who have used pharmaceuticals and over-the-counter remedies, healing these organs takes time. Fortunately, the liver has great regenerative ability, especially when one is less than about 65 years old. We use every method possible to enhance liver functioning. This includes:

a) A clean, healthy diet and pure water to drink, as explained above.

b) A healthful lifestyle, especially going to bed by 9 Pm and lots of rest and sleep. The liver does its main work during rest and sleep. Missing this single factor is often a key as to why some do not succeed in restoring the liver.

c) Nutritional support for the liver includes milk thistle, dandelion root and perhaps other herbal products that are superb. Be careful with some herbs, however, such as burdock root and others, as they are somewhat toxic. They may be used for a short time, but are not for ongoing use as milk thistle and dandelion can be used.

d) Other procedures for the liver are a daily coffee enema, or even two per day for very toxic conditions, colonic irrigation to reduce debris and fermentation and putrefaction in the colon, castor oil packs over the liver and the use of a near infrared lamp sauna.

Using a near infrared sauna on a daily basis, or better twice daily is also very helpful for liver detoxification. Traditional saunas and far infrared saunas may be okay, but do not seem to work as well. Far infrared types may emit harmful electromagnetic frequencies.

e) Attitude change is critical for the liver in some cases. The liver is associated with a "bilious personality". In modern language, this means anger, resentment, hatred and other harmful emotions. For some people, this is the key to their liver regeneration. Meditation, relaxation and forgiveness are thus important for the liver.

f) Other healing modalities may help, especially body work such as Rolfing, acupuncture and acupressure. For instance, we recommend everyone to rub their feet each day. This seems simple and maybe silly, but can have beneficial effects, particularly if one is skilled at it. The technique is easy to learn and to practice.

The kidneys. To restore the kidneys, many of the same items are critical. These include an excellent diet that is balanced for the oxidation type, along with a very healthful lifestyle and a life free of toxic pollutants. Other items include:

a) Herbs for the kidneys. Uva ursi, parsley and other herbs are helpful to a degree. We also use kidney glandular substance with excellent results.

b) Drinking plenty of spring or distilled water is critical for the kidneys. Be sure to drink enough pure water (3 quarts or more daily for most everyone). No other type of water is recommended except spring or steam distilled water. However, drink distilled water for only about three months and no more. After this, it will begin to remove some beneficial minerals.

Strictly avoid reverse osmosis water, "drinking waters", most "purified water" and alkaline waters. Carbon-only filtered tap water is okay and second-best, but not as good in most cases as good spring water. Preferably drink an hour after meals or up to 15 minutes before meals, rather than with meals. Read Water for Drinking for much more on drinking water.

c) Rest is also critical for the kidneys, which are close to and associated with the adrenal glands. This, in Chinese terminology, is related to the kidney meridian, a meridian that is very weak on most people. Rest cannot be overestimated to restore the kidneys and the adrenal glands.

The skin. This is the third most important eliminative organ, and most doctors pay no attention to it whatsoever! In most people, today, including most children, it is toxic or congested and for these reasons quite underactive in its job of eliminating many toxins from the body. This even applies to newborns today. Vaccines affect the skin and can cause it to become less active, as can over dressing infants. Bathing in toxic bath water harms the skin, as can tight clothing and some synthetic clothing. The use of toxic lotions, skin creams, and body care products also harms the skin of many people.

Sauna therapy. Improving the skin requires a lot of work in most cases. Even with two saunas daily, plus all our other efforts, just restoring the skin will take six to twelve months in most adults. Children require less, as their skin is usually in far better condition due to more sweating and fewer toxic exposures. Saunas draw blood to the surface, powerfully stimulate circulation and decongest the internal organs. Infrared saunas penetrate more deeply and are often more comfortable as they work at lower temperatures.

I find the best saunas are those powered by infrared heat lamps. Far infrared saunas are okay, in most cases, but are not as good as a near infrared lamp sauna. Almost all far infrared saunas emit stray electromagnetic fields that affect some people. Steam baths and other procedures such as skin brushing, sitting in hot tubs or others may be used, but are not nearly as good. Sweating during exercise is also not nearly as good, but better than nothing. As an example of what saunas can do, The New York Times recently reported on the success of sauna therapy to help hundreds of New York firemen. They had become ill from the World Trade Tower disaster. No other medical or alternative therapy was able to help these brave men and women to recover their health. Refer to the articles on this site about Sauna Therapy for more information.

The large intestine. This is also an important organ of elimination and one that is in terrible condition in the vast majority of people. Fortunately, it is easier to correct than the skin, liver or kidneys. Diet, of course, plays a critical role in rehabilitating the intestines. Eliminating sugar is most important, even the sugar found in too much fruit or juices. Fiber is critical, as is enough protein for the intestine to rebuild itself. In addition, lifestyle is important and coffee enemas can greatly speed the elimination of toxins from the large intestine and liver that often leads to bowel problems.

Other aids for digestion are other digestive aids such as Betaine Hcl-pepsin, bromelain and others. However, they are not as good. Deep breathing, some exercise and adequate rest and sleep are important for digestive strength as well. Staying warm in winter is important as well.

TOXIC METAL REMOVAL WITH NUTRITIONAL BALANCING

Even with an excellent quality diet, healthful lifestyle, and consistent daily use of near infrared sauna therapy, coffee enemas and short-term use of distilled water for about 6 months, but usually not longer, toxic metal removal at the deepest levels takes a number of years in almost everyone we have encountered. This means that repeated hair mineral analyses keep revealing more and more of the metals coming out of the body through the hair and skin, often for 5 to 10 years.

This is not because nutritional balancing science is slow to remove the toxic metals. I believe it does it faster than any other method of removing toxins from the body such as chelation therapy, herbs, clay baths and other methods. It also does it in a much safer manner.

The reason it takes so long is that nutritional balancing removes many more of the toxic metals, and this is a slow process for the following reasons:

• Toxicity of the metals. They are extremely toxic substances. If they were removed too quickly, they could poison or even kill a person. The body seems to know how to remove them at a pace that is safe, providing we keep balancing the body chemistry and supporting a person the entire time. Otherwise, it just takes longer. Rarely, a person will have a powerful toxic reaction as a heavy metal is released from a storage site, but this is not common.

• Location of the metals, in some instances. Some storage sites of the body are much harder to reach than others due to impaired circulation, or other difficulties such as the blood-brain barrier and others. Toxic metals in the bones, for example, usually take longer to reach as well due to reduced circulation and just the depth or layer of the tissue where they are stored. Sites that have suffered damage and some scarring such as often the ear canals, bronchial, lungs and other tissues may also be harder to regenerate and thus take longer.

• Incorporated into enzymes. Toxic metals are often not just in deposits or floating free in the tissues, although this is true of some of them. These are the easiest to remove. Unfortunately, millions of molecules are replacing essential minerals in enzymes throughout the body. They cannot simply be pulled out with a chelator or anything. The body must very carefully and slowly replace them with enzymes that contain essential minerals. This is a much slower process, but a vital one that slowly increases a person's energy level and restores functioning of all the body organs as well.

• Low vitality. Energy is required to synthesize new enzymes, carry away toxic metals and activate the eliminative organs to remove them completely. Most people, especially when they begin a program, have low cellular energy production that makes this process much slower.

•   Impaired eliminative channels. All toxic metals must be flushed or removed from the body through the so-called eliminative channels or organs such as the liver, kidneys, bowel and skin. Some can be removed through the lungs and else-where but these are the main routes. Most people have very damaged livers, colons and skin, so this slows the process of metal elimination drastically, often for a few years until these organs can be rebuilt and function at their optimum levels.

•   Impaired general nutrition. As ex-plained above, toxic metals must often be replaced by vital minerals in enzymes. One may think that just swallowing some kelp capsules or other supplements and eating well will provide these replacements. However, the body has complex buffering systems, and it will only accept a certain amount of these es-sential minerals at one time. This is even true if one decides to take mineral in intravenously or intramus-cularly. Each mineral must be bound to a mineral transporter to be properly utilized in many instances and the process of demineralizing and nourishing a body thus is a time-consuming process no matter what. If I felt that IV or IM minerals and other nutri-ents were better, I would suggest it but so far I have seen the opposite. Other than very gross demineral-izing of the body, these routes of administering nu-trients seem to do more damage by unbalancing the delicate mineral balance of the body and bypassing the normal buffering systems of the body having to do with food absorption. Exceptions to this principle may exist, but they are not many.

SYMPTOMS WITH TOXIC METAL RE-MOVAL

The elimination of heavy metals, as well as the removal of toxic chemicals and chronic infections, almost always will cause symptoms from time to time. These symptoms are called healing reactions flare-ups, exacerbations, aggravations, crises of Herxheimer reactions in different natural healing arts. They may include energy fluctuations, headaches, skin rashes and other symptoms as well.

Emotional and mental symptoms often occur as well. These include feelings of depression, anxiety, irritability, insomnia or mood swings. All purification symptoms tend to be very temporary. The best way to handle them is to rest more, reduce your nutrition program if you wish and do supportive therapies.

These include extra coffee enemas, drinking distilled water in larger quantities, short, rather than longer sauna therapy sessions, colonic irrigation, Epsom salt baths and others. In almost all cases, this will suffice to move the toxic metals out of the body a little faster and the symptom will disappear.

At times, more vigorous or severe healing reactions occur. Almost any symptom can arise, from a cold or flu to various aches and pains or other types of symptoms.

Usually only supportive, natural methods of care are needed to see a reaction through to completion. However, if you are not sure, always contact a person knowledgeable in healing and purification reactions. For more information, read other articles on this website such as Retracing and Copper Elimination Symptoms.

SYMPTOMS OF THE COMMON TOXIC METALS

SOURCES
Aluminum - cookware, beverages in aluminum cans, tap water, table salt, baking powders, antacids, processed cheese, anti-perspirants, bleached flour, vaccines and perhaps other medications, and occupational exposure. Virtually everyone has too much aluminum in their bodies.

Antimony – found in Flovent, an inhaler used for asthma! Also used in lead-acid batteries, "lead-free" solder, bullets, motor bearings, pewter, some paints and glass, and some microelectronic circuits. It was formerly used in some anti-parasitic drugs.

Antimony is also used in most fire retardants that are required on most furniture, mattresses, cribs and other products. This is severely increasing the prevalence of antimony toxicity in homes and offices.

Arsenic - pesticides, beer, table salt, tap water, paints, pigments, cosmetics, glass and mirror manufacture, fungicides, insecticides, treated wood and contaminated food.

Beryllium - air pollution (burning fossil fuels), manufacture of plastics, electronics, steel alloys and volcanic ash.

Cadmium - cigarettes, (tobacco and marijuana), processed and refined foods, large fish, shellfish, tap water, auto exhaust, plated containers, galvanized pipes, air pollution from incineration and occupational exposure.

Copper - copper water pipes, copper added to tap water, pesticides, swimming in pools, intrauterine devices, vegetarian diets, dental amalgams, nutritional supplements - especially prenatal vitamins, birth control pills, weak adrenal glands and occupational exposure.

Lead - tap water, cigarette smoke, hair dyes, paints, inks, glazes, pesticide residues and occupational exposure in battery manufacture and other industries.

Mercury - dental amalgams, ALL fish (tiny fish are better), ALL shellfish, sea vegetables, some medications such as thiazide diuretics, air pollution, gold mining, and the manufacture of paper, chlorine, adhesives, fabric softeners and waxes. Most everyone has too much mercury in their body today.

Nickel - hydrogenated oils (margarine, commercial peanut butter and shortening), shellfish, air pollution, cigarette smoke, plating and occupational exposure.

SYMPTOMS

Aluminum – Alzheimer's disease, amyotrophic lateral sclerosis, anemia and other blood disorders, colic, fatigue, dental caries, dementia dialactica, hypoparathyroidism, kidney and liver dysfunctions, neuromuscular disorders, osteomalacia and Parkinson's disease.

Antimony – Symptoms are usually chronic. Skin exposure can cause dermatitis. Lung exposure causes irritation and inflammation. Chronic use of Flovent (a drug) appears to keep the hair phosphorus level low. This may indicate impairment of protein biosynthesis.

Arsenic - abdominal pain, abnormal ECG, anorexia, dermatitis, diarrhea, edema, enzyme inhibitor, fever, fluid loss, goiter, hair loss, headache, herpes, impaired healing, interferes with the uptake of folic acid, inhibition of sulfhydryl enzyme systems, jaundice, keratosis, kidney and liver damage, muscle spasms, pallor, peripheral neuritis, sore throat, stomatitis, stupor, vasodilation, vertigo, vitiligo and weakness.

Beryllium - adrenal insufficiency, arthritis, and bone spurs, bursitis, depression, fatigue, osteoporosis and symptoms of slow metabolism.

Cadmium - hypertension, arthritis, diabetes, anemia, arteriosclerosis, impaired bone healing, cancer, cardiovascular disease, cirrhosis, reduced fertility, hyperlipidemia, hypoglycemia, headaches, osteoporosis, kidney disease, schizophrenia and strokes.

Copper - acne, adrenal hyperactivity and/or insufficiency, agoraphobia, allergies, hair loss, anemia, anxiety, arthritis, autism, cancer, chronic candida albicans infection, depression, elevated cholesterol, cystic fibrosis, depression, diabetes, dyslexia, elevated estrogen, failure to thrive, fatigue, fears, fractures of the bones, headaches, heart attacks, hyperactivity, hypertension, hypothyroidism, infections, inflammation, insomnia, iron storage diseases, kidney and liver dysfunctions, decreased libido, multiple sclerosis, nervousness, osteoporosis, panic attacks, premenstrual syndrome, schizophrenia, strokes, tooth decay and vitamin C and other vitamin deficiencies.

Lead - abdominal pain, adrenal insufficiency, anemia, arthritis, arteriosclerosis, attention deficit, back problems, blindness, cancer, constipation, convulsions, deafness, depression, diabetes, dyslexia, epilepsy, fatigue, gout, impaired glycogen storage, hallucinations, hyperactivity, impotency, infertility, inflammation, kidney dysfunction, learning disabilities, diminished libido, migraine headaches, multiple sclerosis, psychosis, thyroid imbalances and tooth decay.

Mercury - adrenal gland dysfunction, alopecia, anorexia, ataxia, bipolar disorder, birth defects, blushing, depression, dermatitis, discouragement, dizziness, fatigue, headaches, hearing loss, hyperactivity, immune system dysfunction, insomnia, kidney damage, loss of self-control, memory loss, mood swings, nervousness, numbness and tingling, pain in limbs, rashes, excessive salivation, schizophrenia, thyroid dysfunction, timidity, tremors, peripheral vision loss and muscle weakness.

Nickel - cancer (oral and intestinal), depression, heart attacks, hemorrhages, kidney dysfunction, low blood pressure, malaise, muscle tremors and paralysis, nausea, skin problems, tetany and vomiting.

***

Chapter 4

Retracing & Healing reactions

WHAT IS RETRACING?

Retracing is a specific type of deep healing that fully restores the anatomy and physiology of a part of the body. The basis for retracing is that as one goes through life, most people do not handle all traumas, infections, injuries and other insults to the body and brain correctly. Instead of moving through them properly until they are fully handled and re-leased, people often become stuck at some point in the process of resolving their traumas. This leaves a trace, a blemish, toxicity, a scar or an unhealed area in the body and/or brain.

The retracing experience or process is one of completing the healing of these blemishes or traumas. Retracing has to do with a wave concept. When one is traumatized by a toxin, an infection, or a mental or emotional situation, ideally one should move through a series of steps – like a wave motion – in order to fully resolve, regenerate, and restore the body and brain.

These steps are:

1. The up part of the wave = the inflammatory response. In this step, the body and/or brain mobilize their forces to fight off and overcome the insult, toxin or situation.

A fight ensues. This is when a child might scream or cry, and it might last half an hour, or as long as it takes to overcome the trauma or insult to the body.

2. The down wave = regeneration. This is a quieter period of time when the body and brain send nutrients to the area to rebuild, restore and regenerate tissue. If the original trauma was mental or emotional, the person might need a hug or a kiss, or just a nap so that the nervous can rebalance and restore itself to equilibrium where it knows it is loved and all is well.

At the end of the down wave phase, one is fully healed and restored, and ready to face the world once again. Retracing is ONLY needed when a person does not complete all these steps in the wave, and instead gets stuck somewhere in the process.

When this occurs, in order to complete the healing process, one must go back into the situation, or metaphorically "revisit the scene of the crime" and process the entire situation correctly. This is what you are doing when you retrace.

It is often somewhat confusing because the original insult, illness or trauma occurred when you were perhaps 2, or 5 or 10 years of age. You may not recall the event at all, or it was suppressed, and often not well understood.

Now you are 25, 40 or perhaps 60 years old, with much greater mental clarity. However, you must go back and re-experience the event as it happened, and finish processing it. This may involve feeling "ill" for a few days or longer, and it may involve retracing and processing emotions and thoughts that were part of the incident.

For more on the stress wave, please read The Stress Wave on this site.

Requirements for the process of retracing.

1. A drastic increase in the vitality or adaptive energy level of the body.

2. Then an old emotional or mental trauma, an infection, or some other blemish or imbalance comes up into waking consciousness for review.

3. One must then re-experience, and process the event properly. This may involve reframing, redoing, re-analyzing or just handling a symptom without panicking. When you do this properly, the symptom or condition resolves and vanishes, and is gone forever.

However, if it is a major infection or mental trauma, it may not all resolve at one time. One may need to resolve part of it at a time, until after several flare-ups it is totally healed, which means you are made whole.

The retracing process is very different from healing or cures that occur with medical drugs, vitamins, herbs, and most other methods of getting rid of symptoms. In the latter, symptoms may go away, but the whole body system is not restored to its previous wholeness.

With medical and holistic "cures", one may become dependent upon a remedy, or there is a residual toxicity in the body due to the remedy, or the remedy masks the symptom. None of these outcomes is the same as completing a wave of regeneration, which is what occurs with the process of retracing.

Retracing is almost unknown and poorly understood in conventional medicine and in holistic medical arts because it rarely occurs with their methods of care. However, it is one of the most important and essential aspects of nutritional balancing science.

WHAT ARE HEALING REACTIONS?

The healing reactions are temporary symptoms that occur as a result of the retracing process. Healing reactions are welcome signs of healing. In fact, if they fail to occur, one knows that a healing method may offer symptomatic relief, but usually it is not as deep or complete as those therapies that cause healing reactions.

Most of the time, healing reactions are mild and may not even be noticed. Once in a while, however, they are annoying and unpleasant. This article will help you handle all types of healing reactions.

PRINCIPLES TO HELP UNDERSTAND HEALING REACTIONS

1. The body will not undertake a healing reaction unless it can see it through to completion. I have found this to be true in at least 95% of healing crises, no matter how vigorous or unusual the symptoms.

2. Due to principle #1 above, reassurance and general supportive measures are usually all that is required, even with an intense purification or healing reaction. These measures are discussed below and include plenty of rest, a simple diet, and keeping a positive attitude.

Fearing these reactions, and reacting with horror or severe anxiety, definitely impairs the body's ability to move through the reaction.

4. A nutritional balancing program causes continuous retracing. Healing occurs fast, and at deep levels, causing this. Therefore, any symptoms during a nutritional balancing program tend to be due to only three possibilities:

A) The program needs updating.

B) It is a healing reaction.

C) One is not following the program correctly. The usual way this occurs is that one is not eating enough cooked vegetables. These are absolutely needed to assist the body to remove toxic metals and chemicals, and to re-nourish the body.

TYPES OF HEALING REACTIONS DURING NUTRITIONAL BALANCING PROGRAMS

Fairly common reactions during a nutritional balancing program:

- Fatigue

- Anxiety

- Colds and flus

- Skin rashes

- Sleep disturbances

- Bowel disturbances such as constipation or diarrhea, at times

- Testicular pain in men

- Changes in the menstrual period in young women

- Ear symptoms

- Throat symptoms

- Chest wall pain

- Liver/gall bladder pain

- Solar plexus pain

- Other aches and pains

- Spinal release (discussed below)

- Fevers or night sweats

Rarer reactions:

- Appendix retracing

- Nodules and lumps

- Bleeding

- Breathing difficulty

However, they are almost always benign and due to:

a) Retracing an infection or other condition.

b) Toxin elimination.

c) A need to update the program.

Most symptoms during a nutritional balancing go away on their own in few days to a week, and do not require any medical intervention. If any symptom persists or is bothersome, always check with your practitioner.

Types of healing reactions:

A. REMOVAL REACTIONS (4 of them):

1. Healing (removal) of an infection. This was noted by medical doctors (Jarisch and Herxheimer) over 100 years ago. Most adults have at least a dozen chronic infections.

Common locations are the sinuses, ears, eyes, teeth, gums, throat, skin, bronchial, lungs, stomach, intestines, liver, and colon. Even young children and babies have a number of infections that will flare up temporarily as they become acute and heal.

More serious infections will flare up, then diminish, and may flare up again several times until they are removed completely. Some of these clients had experienced ear infections.

Antibiotic therapy kills most bacteria, but it does not heal the body tissues. As a result, some infections remain and fester in a chronic way. Some antibiotic residues also remain in the body for years, altering the normal intestinal flora and causing many other problems.

For these reasons, please take antibiotics only as a last resort. Natural products are usually effective. For more, please read Beyond Antibiotics on this site.

Viruses. Many chronic infections are viral. As the body's vitality improves, they retrace and disappear. They can include herpes and other sexually-transmitted diseases.

Parasites. There are over 300 species of parasites, and infection is common. Liver flukes are especially widespread. Many of our clients report seeing dead parasites in the toilet during a nutritional balancing program.

No drugs, herbs or other anti-parasitic remedies are needed to remove parasites with a nutritional balancing program. These remedies are all somewhat toxic, so it is best to avoid them all.

2. Removal of a toxic metal. Today, everyone has lots of toxic metals in their body. Children are born with them, and they are in the air, water, food and items we touch every day. Three dozen toxic metals will come out of the body using a nutritional balancing program. They will come out in the body's own order and its own timing.

Toxic metals are usually in compounds or molecules. Some of these are more difficult for the body to eliminate than others. One metal may come out for a few months. Then, another one may come out. Then the previous metal may come out again for another few months, perhaps in a different compound. So the process of removing them is lengthy and complex.

Repeated hair testing sometimes reveals the process, but there are metals that are not tested, and the metals are removed by many routes – the colon, the skin, the liver, and the lungs. Fortunately, we don't need to know which are coming out to adjust the nutritional balancing program.

3. Removal of a toxic chemical. Many people have been exposed to solvents, pesticides, paints, and

other toxic chemicals. Some are aware of the exposure, but most people have little memory of the incident.

Symptoms that occur as the chemicals are eliminated may include strange odors, odd tastes, rashes, liver or kidney pain, diarrhea, constipation, or other symptoms. These chemicals are acquired in utero, or afterwards from food, water, air or from contact with many household and industrial products.

4. Removal of bad quality tissue. A common one is intestinal lining. Clients occasionally think that a piece of twisted intestinal lining in the toilet is a parasite. Removal of toxic tissue occasionally causes weight loss that worries our clients.

5. Removal of a mental or emotional "toxins" and traumas. Most people have experienced traumas of a mental or emotional type. These may be brought to consciousness for processing and removal. It is an amazing aspect of a nutritional balancing program.

It is due to better mental clarity, and improvements in memory and vitality. Also, the removal of toxic metals can sometimes free one of long-held emotions such as anger or fear. Some of clients are quite upset when they suddenly begin thinking or dreaming about their divorce, death of child years ago, or some other issue. However, deep healing of the body and mind requires that such traumas be exposed, processed and removed.

METABOLIC SHIFTS

1. A change in the oxidation rate or oxidation type. This is very common. Slowing of the oxidation rate may cause one to feel more tired or depressed. If the oxidation rate increases, one may feel more energetic or perhaps just more irritable.

If the oxidation type changes, then the nutritional balancing program must be adjusted, or one will feel that the program is making one worse – and it is. Rarely, the oxidation rate and type fluctuate up and down, over and over again, confusing things. Fortunately, this is not common.

2. A shift in the sodium/potassium ratio. This is important because it, too, necessitates a change in the nutritional balancing supplement program. Zinc is needed if the ratio is above 2.5, while Limcomin is needed if the ratio drops below 2.5. Keeping this ratio near its ideal level of 2.5 is very important to feel well and to keep any healing reaction going through to completion.

3. A shift into or out of other mineral patterns. This occurs continuously during the retracing process. They are necessary, at times, to remove toxic metals, to heal infections, and to process mental and emotional traumas.

For example, the body might temporarily shift into a four lows mineral pattern, a bowl pattern, or any of two dozen others. This is perfectly normal as part of retracing.

4. Other biochemical shifts. Many are possible, such as changes in gland and hormone secretion, changes in the intestinal flora, more bile secretion, or a change in body temperature, bowel habits, blood sugar or blood pressure. These are all normal and to be expected.

Abnormal blood readings. A problem our clients have is that these changes often upset routine blood tests. They easily cause abnormal thyroid, liver and other test readings.

5. A structural shift. This is caused by a change in muscle tension, changes in the ligaments and tendons, adjustment of the spine or other bones, more nerve energy flowing to certain areas, or some other mechanism.

Spinal release. A number of people who follow a nutritional balancing program experience a spinal release healing reaction. This is a more extensive change in the bone structure. It often begins in the lumbar and sacral areas, and slowly moves up the spine to the thoracic and cervical areas. It may be caused by more etheric energy flowing through the spinal nerves. It can cause annoying temporary symptoms of back pain or sciatic pain.

The spine relaxes and lets go in an uneven way, giving rise to the pain until the back finally balances out. Chiropractic care is often necessary for a while. Other helpful modalities are the spinal twist exercise, foot reflexology, and the red heat lamp shined on the back. The spinal release reaction can take a year or more to complete.

UNUSUAL HEALING REACTIONS DURING A NUTRITIONAL BALANCING PROGRAM

The following three types of pain and tenderness bother some people during the program. All are benign and will go away, but they are worth discussing so as not to be concerned.

Pain in the liver and gall bladder area. This occurs in some people on the program. It has to do with the liver acupuncture meridian, which becomes stressed as the liver eliminates many toxins.

The liver meridian runs down the front of the body from the right shoulder through the right nipple and gall bladder to the right leg crease. From there it turns around and goes up the back through the inner part of the shoulder blade and back up to the right shoulder. In some women, the right bra shoulder strap makes the pain much worse and not wearing a bra helps. This pain is not a cause for alarm. It is not a disease. It will slowly subside if one stays with the nutritional balancing program. However, it can take several years or longer to go away.

Coffee enemas are always helpful to speed healing of this meridian. Also helpful is opening the central channel or Conception Vessel in acupuncture terminology. Actually, this type of pain and tenderness can be helpful. It tends to make a person stay with their health program.

Pain and tenderness in the solar plexus. This is also somewhat common during a nutritional balancing program. Clients often think it is stomach pain, gastritis, or an ulcer. However, it is none of these. It has to do with the third energy center and with an etheric gathering point or terminal that is located slightly above the umbilicus or belly button. It is a very positive sign!

It is not a problem, and it will slowly go away if one stays on the program. Interestingly, having a lot of children helps with congestion in this area. Those who have not been parents usually feel this reaction the most. For more, please read Third Center Pain on this site.

Chest wall pain. This also occurs, at times, during a nutritional balancing program. It is caused by tension in the intercostal muscles. For more about it, please read Chest Wall Pain.

Burning pain upon urination. Once in a while, a client reports burning pain in the urethra and bladsder area upon urination. This can occur in children, at times, as well.

The cause is either retracing of an old bladder infection or the release of an irritating toxin through the kidneys and into the urine. Retracing an old urinary tract infection is often helped by taking vitamin A – up to 20,000 iu daily for adults and less for children. Genital baths- 5 or 6 daily – are easy to do and also excellent for this symptom. Rubbing the bladder reflex area of both feet (outside, below the ankle bone, near the bottom of the foot but on the side, not the bottom) is also excellent, at times.

For the release of a toxin through the kidneys and bladder, drink more water, and perhaps take an Epsom salt bath – but no more than 3 baths per week. Both are benign, and tend to pass quickly. If it continues and is annoying, reduce the supplement program and it will likely slow down the elimination and thus the pain or burning sensation will diminish. Eventually, it will pass when the toxin is completely eliminated.

MENTAL AND EMOTIONAL PURIFICATION SYMPTOMS

These may include irritability, anxiety, fears, anger, depression, and feelings of panic, brain fogginess, or others. Long-forgotten memories occasionally surface, or one may have unusual dreams as the brain processes traumas or incidents from the past. Unusual dreams are not uncommon. In fact, symptoms may include almost anything. Most healing reactions are mild and pass quickly.

HANDLING PHYSICAL HEALING REAC- TIONS

In general, the body will not undertake a healing reaction unless it can see it through. Most important is to support the body, allowing it to proceed with minimal interference. At times, one may speed up a reaction so it will end sooner. Other times, one may slow down a reaction to lessen the severity of symptoms. Basic support for reactions is:

1. Lately, many clients have been progressing faster on their nutritional balancing program. Staying on an incorrect program can cause many symptoms! What appears to be a healing reaction can simply be that the body chemistry has changed, and the nutritional balancing supplements, and perhaps the diet, need to be updated.

If you have checked and your program is good, then:

2. Rest lying down as much as possible. Also, reduce stress and strain. Conserve energy for healing. Reduce mental as well as physical activity. Breathing deeply and slowly is very calming for the nervous system.

3. Eat lightly. Digestion is an extra stress during healing reactions. If one is very uncomfortable, it may be best to skip a meal. One may no-

tice that symptoms subside after eating a meal. The meal is not making one better. Energy must be diverted from healing to digest the meal, so symptoms temporarily diminish while one digests.

While drinking adequate water is important during healing reactions, guzzling extra water is usually not helpful.

4. Discontinue most nutritional supplements until a reaction passes. Reactions will proceed without most supplements. Some can impair the healing process. See below for exceptions.

5. Shorten sauna sessions. Continuing with long sauna sessions can intensify a healing reaction. If the liver is being overloaded with toxins, this may not be desirable. It may be best to cease using a sauna or reduce the frequency and duration of sessions until the reaction passes. On the other hand, for clearing an infection, healing a wound or injury or certain other conditions, continuing or even increasing sauna sessions may get it over with faster.

In general, during a healing reaction, 10-15 minute sessions eight times per day are better than long sessions. These are less debilitating in the midst of a healing reaction. When reactions occur, it helps greatly to call and speak with someone familiar with sauna therapy and healing reactions.

6. Other detoxification procedures are often helpful. Besides more short sauna sessions, other procedures include coffee enemas, chiropractic,

and foot reflexology. Enemas are excellent and perhaps essential if one feels constipated and toxic. Chiropractic and related therapies may also be helpful.
Be careful, however, to get references and make sure
anyone you visit is completely reputable.

7. Call your nutritional balancing
practitioner if you are unsure how to handle a reaction. Nutritional balancing is not a do-it-yourself
program. When going through a healing reaction,
your judgment is usually not good. So please contact
your nutritional balancing consultant or doctor. Do
not just try to solve things yourself. This is a hard
and fast rule.

8. Use care in discussing healing reactions with physicians and others unfamiliar with
them. Healing symptoms can easily be misinterpret-
ed as illness. This is a common problem. Unless the
doctor, friend or family member understands, costly
tests and toxic medication may be recommended.
Medication can complicate reactions and is rarely
effective. Reactions will usually proceed in spite of it.

OTHER SUPPORTIVE MEASURES

Watch your attitude. It has been ob-
served during this healing person with negative attitude becomes too fearful with a healing reaction; this
makes it more difficult to move through. So, if possible, relax as much as possible and attempt to be
grateful for this healing action of the body. I know

this is difficult, at times, but a positive attitude is extremely helpful for all healing.

For toxic reactions in general: As toxins are mobilized and eliminated, one may experience headaches, rashes, pain, dizziness, abdominal discomfort and other symptoms. In addition to the general ideas above, more coffee enemas are wonderful for most detoxification reactions of this type. In addition, adding milk thistle and dandelion root to your nutritional balancing program may help.

Nausea is usually due to congestion of the liver due to toxin removal. More coffee enemas, up to four per day, are often helpful. Two coffee enemas can be taken back to back in the morning, and two back to back in the afternoon. This is a powerful combination, and this can be continued for a week or even a month or more, if needed.

In an extreme case, one can induce vomiting if extreme nausea is present. Drink salt water first, so the stomach is not empty. Lying down and remaining quiet for half an hour or more is often very beneficial.

SUPPORT FOR INFECTIONS

Retracing infections is often a bit scary, as one can develop fever, rashes, dizziness and other disturbing symptoms. However, if a person is following a nutritional balancing program, most infections, no matter how vigorous they seem, are benign and ideally should never be suppressed with drugs, high-dose vitamin C, or other remedies. Herbs such as Echinacea, golden seal and astragalus, are okay. At times, colloidal silver is helpful.

Always make sure that one's temperature does not rise above about 103-104 F. If it becomes higher, ways to lower it naturally include sponging the body with cool water and a coffee enema or two will almost always lower a fever. This will have to be repeated every few hours, but that is okay.

Also, be sure you are well-hydrated when fever is present, as the body can easily become dehydrated. Drink water, and not tea or juice.

Common sites of chronic infections are the sinuses, ears, eyes, throat, bronchial, lungs, intestines, kidneys and bladder. Most people have dozens of chronic infections that commonly flare up as they are healed. They go from chronic to acute, and are then eliminated. This is the reverse order in which they took hold in the body. Here are some simple and safe supportive therapies that are excellent for retracing infections.

Coffee enemas. These are excellent to help one move through any infection or fever. Up to four per day is fine.

Heat. Heat activates the immune system and may disable or even kill some microorganisms. For this reason, sauna use is excellent to help heal some chronic infections. Do not continue with sauna therapy if it just irritates the body, which occasionally occurs. It can be confusing, however, because at times the seeming irritation can be a healing process.

The light of the reddish heat lamp and the heat of the sauna definitely upset most parasites, which is a type of 'cold' or 'yin' infection. One can expose an area of chronic infection to more infrared as this can speed healing in some cases. This works very well on the sinuses, for example, and can work well with parasites in the intestinal tract or elsewhere in the body.

Another excellent idea is to shine one or more red heat lamps on the thymus gland area, which is the middle of the chest or breast bone. Do this for 30 minutes at a time, twice or three times daily. This may also speed up healing.

Diet. Eat lightly. Drink plenty of spring water. Eat less, especially if you are not too hungry. Never eat a lot when sick. Infection remedies when retracing. Check with your consultant about taking any of these remedies, as they will be indicated sometimes, but not others.

They include:

Limcomin. This is a product from Endomet Laboratories that contains some zinc, copper, vitamins A and C, and a little magnesium and vitamin B6. It is designed to support the immune response, and often works extremely well. Adults can take up to 6 tablets three times daily. Children need less depending on their size and weight.

Vitamin A (and not beta carotene). This is one of the most used natural remedies in nutritional balancing science. It strengthens mucus membranes and has other positive effects upon the immune response, so it is helpful for many infections of all kinds. Adults usually need about 25,000 to 50,000 iu per day for 5 days or so. The natural vitamin A from fish oil is somewhat better than the synthetic form, called retinyl palmitate.

Colloidal silver. I prefer the following brands, although other may work well, too. Arabesque, Endomet, Sovereign Silver and Live Silver. However, other brands are sometimes very good, too. The usual dose for a low-potency product for an adult is about 1 tablespoon three times daily, taken by itself, at least 15 minutes away from all food and all beverages before and after taking it. It may also be applied locally by sniffing it, inhaling it or putting it on the skin or a drop in an ear, for example.

Zinc. This important mineral by itself is usually not indicated during healing reactions because it lowers the tissue sodium level, which is usually low to begin with. However, in combination with copper, manganese, vitamin A and vitamin C, in the product called Limcomin, it is extremely helpful, at times.

Vitamin C. A little vitamin C boosts adrenal activity and helps raise the Na/K ratio. It also has some immune-boosting ability. Warning: As a general rule, do not use high-dose vitamin C when following a nutritional balancing program. It upsets body chemistry, lowers copper, is too yin and is not needed. Warning: Especially avoid extra vitamin C if a person is a fast oxidizer or is in a four lows pattern because these people need copper badly, and vitamin C lowers copper in the body. Vitamin A is generally much better than vitamin C for retracing reactions.

Herbs such as Echinacea, golden seal, astragalus. These are used, at times, but I find they are not as helpful today, for some reason, as in the past.

Bee propolis. This is occasionally helpful for those following a nutritional balancing program.

Lifestyle. Rest lying down as much as possible. Any infection that persists for more than several days may not be a healing reaction. In this case, consult a knowledgeable practitioner as infections can become serious threats to one's health.

SUPPORT FOR OTHER COMMON RETRACING SYMPTOMS

For Pain in the Liver Area (which is common during a nutritional balancing program):

1. Rub the feet in the liver reflex area and on the top of both feet in the webbing between the first and second toes

2. Extra coffee enemas are often excellent.

3. You can also try taking extra ox bile and pancreatin (such as GB-3 by Endomet Labs).

4. You can add silymarin or milk thistle tincture and/or dandelion tincture. The tincture is often better than dry tablets. For adults, one can take up to 20 drops three times a day or up to 3 capsules three times per day of a standardized product.

For pain in the kidneys or ureters:

1. Drink extra water, up to one quart extra per day.

2. Distilled water for a few days is sometimes remarkably helpful.

3. Stinging nettles may be helpful, up to 20 drops three times/day of a standardized extract.

For Diarrhea: Elimination of antibiotics, metals or toxic chemicals may cause diarrhea. Rest plenty and eat lightly. Be sure to drink enough water to avoid dehydration. Avoid all fruit and all sweets!

Six charcoal tablets, three times per day will help absorb toxins.

In India, we use turmeric, garlic, pepper, sliced ginger in regular meal. Well-cooked garlic or 15 garlic capsules daily may be needed if one is releasing parasites. Eat lightly of non-fibrous, non-irritating foods such as rice, other grains, chicken and cooked vegetables until diarrhea passes. Severe diarrhea that persists requires intervention. Otherwise one may lose vital electrolytes and become dehydrated.

For Emotional Reactions: Emotional traumas deeply held need to be brought to consciousness to be released. When emotions or negative thoughts arise, allow one to feel them without suppressing or wallowing in the feelings. I have observed this technique in Vipassana as well formulated by Buddha.

Doing more of the Roy Masters meditation exercise can be most helpful, as can the physical procedures such as coffee enemas, near infrared lamp sauna sessions, rubbing the feet, and the others.

Observe feelings from as neutral a viewpoint as possible. It is very helpful to talk with someone supportive to gain added perspective. Feelings will generally pass, washing over one like ocean waves. Vigorous exercise can slow emotional reactions. Extra rest and sleep will help them pass more quickly.

Many people learned well to suppress their feelings and have great difficulty expressing them. One may become afraid of one's own buried feelings. These people benefit from allowing themselves to cry, scream or otherwise express that which they feel. If this seems embarrassing, one can close the bedroom door or go sit in a car.

For Nervousness And Anxiety: Elimination of stored caffeine, theophylline, diet pills or other stimulant substances can cause temporary feelings of anxiety as they are released. These will pass without requiring supportive therapy. Extreme fatigue or copper elimination can also cause feelings of anxiety.

If a feeling is very intense or persistent, nutritional supplements of calcium, magnesium, zinc, TMG (trimethylglycine) and/or ICMN (a product containing choline, inositol, methionine and niacinamide) may have a calming effect.

One may take up to 2500 mg of calcium, 1500 mg of magnesium, 100 mg of zinc, 4000 mg of TMG, and/or 1000 mg of choline, inositol, methionine and niacinamide in a 24-hour period. Sometimes one of these works better than another.

Resting, deep, slow breathing, calming herbs, massage, foot reflexology and other natural therapies may be helpful as well.

For Weight Loss or Gain: During nutritional balancing programs, weight may fluctuate. Weight gain may occur if the body retains water to buffer toxins that are being eliminated. Weight loss may occur even in a thin person as damaged tissue is broken down. One often will go through periods of greater tissue breakdown followed by periods of re-building. Shifts in glandular activity may temporari-ly cause weight gain or loss.

Most shifts in weight are not a cause for concern. In some cases, eating more or fewer cal-ories may assist in balancing weight during a detoxi-fication program. Usually, however, the nutritional balancing program needs to take its course and weight will normalize after several months to several years, depending on the toxicity of the body.

To Slow Healing Reactions: Accord-ing to Dr. Paul Eck's research, taking lecithin gran-ules can help slow the elimination of toxic metals and chemicals. Do not take lecithin otherwise. Taking aspirin, Tylenol, tranquilizers or other over the-counter remedies is never recommended.

Crutches are items or methods that just sup-port a person while he or she goes through the pain or discomfort of a healing reaction or retracing. Pushers support one, but they also move one faster through one's issues or healing reactions, and there-fore are even better than crutches. However, pushers often cause more intense temporary pain or other symptoms, which some people do not like.

HEALING REACTIONS IN THE TEETH

These are among the most common healing reactions that occur during a nutritional balancing program. Commonly, pain, sensitivity, loose teeth or an abscess will appear suddenly in a tooth or gum area, with no warning. An X-ray will show what looks like decay, inflammation or an abscess.

In most cases, a dentist will recommend removal of the tooth, root canal treatment, antibiotics, or something else fairly drastic. However, in almost all cases, if one just persists on a nutritional balancing program, the entire episode will pass, leaving no residual damage or other effects.

STRUCTURAL RETRACING

To get well, some people must change the configuration or shape of their structure. It can be their cranial structure, their posture and their spine, or other structural components of the body.

For this purpose, nutritional balancing is superb. In addition, usually the person will need chiropractic care, perhaps for an extended period of years. Bodywork such as Rolfing or Structural Integration may also be helpful. Techniques such as Feldenkreis work and others may also be helpful.

Here is an example of this type of retracing. An elderly man (age 72), who had been a client for several years, suddenly developed a frozen shoulder. He woke up one morning and could not raise his right arm. He visited his medical doctor, who took an X-ray and told him there was a lot of arthritis in the shoulder joint and he should have a shoulder joint replacement as soon as possible.

Finally, he met a nutrition expert. He told him that he had arthritis and it was probably some kind of healing reaction. He was referred to an excellent chiropractor. Within two visits, the shoulder joint unlocked, and was as good as new.

This case exemplifies a problem with x-rays when one is following a nutritional balancing program. The x-ray showed inflammation and the doctor assumed it was caused by arthritis, as there were symptoms of pain and immobility, as well. However, healing reactions always produce a different kind of inflammation that heals the body. However, it often shows up exactly the same as inflammation due to degeneration of a joint. This is very confusing for doctors and our clients and practitioners, alike.

IS IT RETRACING OR A WORSENING OF HEALTH?

At times, reactions are not due to healing and indicate a worsening of a health condition. This happened to the author when he followed a vegetarian diet for a few years. One reads about retracing, and just assumes that any symptom that arises is a healing or retracing reaction.

It can be vitally important to know if a reaction is due to healing or a worsening of a condition. Answering the five questions below can help one to know which is occurring.

1. Was the person following a nutritional balancing program, including diet, rest, supplements and the proper application of the sauna? Healing reactions occur most often when the body is given all that it needs. If the complete program is followed fairly strictly, the reaction is likely due to healing.

However, if a person is not following the program, or on a different regimen, then it is more likely that it is not a healing reaction. Also, if one is terminally ill, it may not be a healing reaction.

2. Was one feeling better before the reaction occurred? Healing reactions require energy. One's energy level often increases until sufficient to initiate a reaction. Thus, a reaction can occur and often does just when one is feeling stronger. If one

had been feeling worse, the reaction is less likely due to healing, however.

3. Have the symptom occurred in the past? Often, old symptoms or conditions recur during healing reactions. If one experienced the symptom in even the distant past, it is more likely, though not always, due to healing.

4. Are the symptoms unusual? Healing reactions often produce odd symptom pictures. One might develop a sore throat or flu without fatigue. This occurs when one is really not ill, though one may develop some features of an illness.

5. How long have symptoms lasted? Healing reactions usually do not last long. They may be vigorous but end in a few hours or at most about a week. If a reaction or flare-up lasts more than several weeks, it may be a worsening of one's condition.

This one is tricky, however, because a deep-seated physical or emotional problem may take weeks or months to retrace completely in a few cases. Look to the other questions for more clarity, or do hair analyses retest to gain more insight as to what is going on.

THE PSYCHOLOGY OF HEALING REACTIONS

Healing reactions are often accompanied by psychological shifts. This is an interesting area of study in nutritional balancing science. Changes in perception, cognition, and rate of processing of information may occur.

Physically-linked Reactions: Some emotional toxins are linked to physical toxins and impaired body chemistry. An unhealthy body sends negative messages to the brain. These may be experienced as feelings of fear, anxiety or unworthiness.

Toxic metals can directly affect neurotransmitters and parts of the brain associated with anger, fear and other emotions. Iron, for example, is known to settle in the amygdala, an area of the brain associated with anger.

As physical toxins are eliminated, emotional states will change. As health improves, the body sends positive messages to the brain. For example, an emotional "crisis" may occur as it becomes more difficult to hold on to negative feelings and beliefs. A related cause of a "crisis" is when cognition and perception improve to a point that a person can no longer continue thinking the same improper or false way as before.

Energy-related Reactions: Though often not taught in psychology, energy is required to feel feelings, even to feel a depression. Many times, a mineral analysis has revealed a pattern associated with depression. The client, however, denied the feeling. After weeks or months on a healing program, the client called and may blame me or the healing program for causing feelings of depression.

In fact, the healing program merely enhanced the client's energy and awareness. The client began to feel what had previously been inaccessible or suppressed. Once the feelings surface, they usually resolve quickly on their own. The brain, like the body, is self-healing provided it functions correctly.

For a psychological view of this phenomenon, I recommend a few older psychology books, Arthur Janov's The Primal Scream and The Primal Revolution. Enhanced energy due to natural therapies causes the brain to function better. Clarity of thinking, memory and awareness often improve. This assists one to question beliefs about oneself and about the world. More capable of understanding oneself, one lets go of false beliefs and destructive behaviors.

Completion Reactions: Incompletely healed traumas leave emotional residues. Small children often cry hard when they fall down. They 'work through' the trauma in ten minutes and soon are laughing as if nothing happened. This is the proper way to handle a trauma. If energy is low or if healing is interrupted for some other reason, a residue of the experience remains and one develops fears or other neuroses. As energy and cognition improve, one often spontaneously heals residues of unhealed traumas.

Decompensation Reactions: Certain attitudes and behaviors are compensations for ill health or low energy. As health improves, these are no longer needed and may disappear suddenly. A surprising shift may occur, often accompanied by an insight about oneself or about the world.

Sometimes an emotional toxin is a major stumbling block that stops the healing process until the client is willing to address it. Psychotherapy or other healing modalities may be required. Body work and other therapies can also be excellent to work with emotional wounds that retard healing.

Simple adjustment reactions. These are common and involve a simple replacement of a toxic mineral with a more physiological mineral, or the correction of a simple enzyme system of the body. Another simple reaction or adjustment is the improvement in a glandular or organ activity.

Past Life Retracing. Some people believe in reincarnation – which the soul does not die and inhabits successive bodies, or has multiple lives on earth or elsewhere.

Indeed, some healing reactions, especially among babies and young children, are so bizarre that one must wonder if there is not some truth to the idea of reincarnation and that the soul of a person may need to go back, so to speak, and repent, undo or redo some aspect of a prior physical existence.

To accomplish this type of deep retracing, one generally needs to take a heavier supplement program. Also, the person must follow the diet carefully. At times, one must do the extra procedures such as the light sauna therapy, coffee enemas, foot reflexology and the daily spinal twist. This spinal twist is known as makarasana by Dr. Vethathiri.

"ARMORING UP" PATTERN RELATED TO HEALING REACTIONS

A very interesting pattern seen on retest hair mineral analyses is called armoring up. It consists of a reduction in the readings of some of the toxic metals and nutrient minerals that were already too low so that they now fall into a poor eliminator range, or go deeper into this range.

Armoring up pattern seems to be related to a healing reaction. It is somewhat akin to putting on your armor in order to handle certain old traumas or other old situations.

A very interesting part of this process is that if a person can take enough TMG or trimethylglycine, then armoring up during healing reactions usually does not occur. Armoring up often only occurs, in other words, in those people who do not take about 3000 mg of TMG daily.

The usual reason for this is that the TMG brings up their emotional issues – usually anger toward men - although I do not know why this particular emotion is related to the use of TMG. Most of those unable to take the full amount of TMG are women, but there are some men, as well, and in all cases, so far, the issue is related to men, not to women. TMG is a methyl donor, but it may have other actions as well related to SAM-e, methionine metabolism, homocysteine metabolism, taurine metabolism, and more. This is an interesting research area. For more, please read Armoring Up Pattern on this site.

HEALING REACTIONS ON BLOOD TESTS

Some clients go to medical or other doctors seeking help for a healing reaction. These doctors run blood tests and are often surprised and upset with the results. Common imbalances seen on blood tests during healing reactions are:

- Low thyroid hormone levels, or elevated TSH.

- Slightly elevated liver enzymes due to liver irritation.
- Low sodium and/or chloride levels, due perhaps to kidney irritation.

- Slight macrocytic anemia in a few cases. This can be due to an elimination of toxic iron, which damages some red blood cells. It is actually a slight hemolytic anemia, not pernicious anemia although it appears the same on blood tests.

- Elevated ferritin if the body is eliminating iron or manganese.

None of these imbalances are a cause for alarm, but many doctors do not understand healing reactions, so they may react badly and want more tests, drug or hormone therapy, or other measures to correct the blood tests. In fact, if an abnormal blood or urine test is due to retracing, if one just waits a few weeks to a month, most blood tests will begin to normalize by themselves without a need for more tests or any medical or other type of therapy.

EXTENDED HEALING REACTIONS

While most healing reactions do not last more than a few days or a week, some will persist for a month or up to a year. These are often much deeper healing processes that cannot be resolved quickly. These are among the most difficult reactions to handle because one can easily doubt that anything positive is occurring.

DISCUSSING HEALING REACTIONS

Forewarned, most people handle healing reactions well. One should look forward to reactions as they are evidence of deep healing. Always call someone knowledgeable if 1) you are not sure what is going on, 2) you are concerned or worried, 3) any reaction becomes severe such as a high fever, or 4) a reaction continues for more than a few days.

These healing reactions can be vigorous, but rarely dangerous. Always use common sense, however. Rarely, medical intervention is needed, but certainly not often. Taking medical drugs such as antibiotics and aspirin or others can prolong the reaction or even turn it into a dangerous situation.

METAPHYSICAL ASPECTS OF RETRACING

This is usually part of any healing technique. For example, if you fast or take one meal a day, your body will go through a lot of changes in the metabolic routine for good reasons. Your body will absorb nutrients from the atmosphere. Typically, as your body becomes lighter, healthier with increased energy levels, then it becomes possible to dive deep into psyche. Hence, first your precipitated emotions come out of conscious mind, then the sub-conscious layer, one after the other. These wounds will open up from the sub-conscious to the conscious mind. The best way to handle the situation is to remain calm, unaffected by the past emotions. You must develop ability to be simple aware, alert and witness without partying to it. You should witness the events in sequence without being subjected to the emotional state of mind, thus resulting in healing these wounds.

With nutritional balancing, the job of the practitioner is to just keep balancing and supporting the body and it will automatically retrace and heal hundreds of old wounds, injuries, infections and much more by itself when the conditions are fulfilled to keep enhancing the homeostasis, vitality and nutrition of the body. It is quite an amazing process to behold, although it can be annoying and even scary, at times. This has something to do with a concept called Etheric Reset.

RETRACING IN OTHER HEALING ARTS

The healing reaction resembles bacterial sepsis and can occur after initiation of antibacterial, such as penicillin or tetracycline, for the treatment of louse-borne relapsing fever (80-90% of patients) and in tick-borne relapsing fever (30-40%). An association has been found between the release of heat-stable proteins from spirochetes and the reaction.

Typically, the death of these bacteria and the associated release of endotoxins or lipoproteins occur faster than the body can remove the substances (my italics). It usually manifests within a few hours of the first dose of antibiotic as fever, chills, rigor, hypotension, headache, tachycardia, hyperventilation, vasodilation with flushing, myalgia (muscle pain), exacerbation of skin lesions and anxiety.

The intensity of the reaction indicates the severity of inflammation. Reaction commonly occurs within two hours of drug administration, but is usually self-limiting.

HEALING REACTIONS IN OTHER HEALING ARTS

In adjusting the spine and stretching tissue that has been shortened for many years, it is usually not possible to avoid discomfort and flare-ups. The flare-up can be seen as a good thing because it tends to corroborate our diagnosis and it tells us that we are in the right place. As the chiropractic care continues, pain and discomfort associated with it tends to diminish."

In psychology and psychoanalysis, these reactions are called the catharsis.

The term catharsis has been adopted by modern psychotherapy, particularly Freudian psychoanalysis, to describe the act of expressing, or more accurately, experiencing the deep emotions often associated with events in the individual's past which had originally been repressed or ignored, and had never been adequately addressed or experienced.

Thus, the concept of healing reactions or retracing is not new, nor is it esoteric or unknown.

***

Chapter 5

Epilogue

Your destiny is not made. Indeed, it is in your hands if you believe. There is one thing left called 'HOPE' if you want to survive. By being more aware, we can address all these health related issues before it appears as diseases. As the saying goes, 'Prevention is better than cure', Today, it is even more relevant than before as you'd need to take corrective actions to heal yourself.

The world has become increasingly polluted, inorganic in almost every wake of life and greed for money is driving all sorts of non-sense in the name of rapid Industrialization. Hence, you should take care of yourself and family to ensure that you're able to lead a healthy life with good life span of > 80 years.

You've read the importance of combining yogic practices with key balancing methods of nutrition as described. This is the not the end, it is a new beginning to alleviate yourself from all maladies and a final cure from all ailments. STOP taking all allopath medications, immediately find out nutrition program that would suit you combined with yogic practices described in this book.

Point that Dr. Wilson is trying to prove is that Nutritional balancing can help you alleviate from all deficiencies in body, mind. It is true, 'food is medicine' as described in the Hindu literature and it is found in many instances of ancient scriptures. Hence, in Hinduism, rajas gunas, which are personality traits of angles are influenced by satvic food (vegie) was considered to be the food of angels and gods, whilst tamas gunas influenced by non-vegetarian food that was treated as enabling demonic attitude in you. Indeed, there is a relevance to it as food becomes your body, mind. It induces bio-magnetism at metaphysical level of mind. It is apparent that what you eat is eventually what you'd become. You might have observed the characteristics of an elephant vis-à-vis a tiger. The difference in traits of animal kingdom between carnivores and herbivores is clear. Hence, do not consume animal food for protein. You will get required nutrition in egg, which is rich in protein and it can be considered as a vegetarian diet along with vegetables, pulses, rice, millets and wheat etc.

If you consume red-meat regularly, rest assured of heart attack in mid-forties. Your metabolism is based on good balanced nutrition. It is interesting to analyze toxic metals buried in your bones, brain and hair. Dr. Wilson has tried to factor each of these toxic metals in the body as a major cause of all illness, fatigue etc. It's obvious some of these toxins are caused due to pollution and toxic metals in food, air etc.

Last but not least, wellness is your birthright! You have every right to defend yourself and enjoy the ultimate freedom by practicing yoga, meditation and introspection exercises. You've been abused by the respective governments in the name of health insurance, allopathic etc. Most of these so called diseases as they named 'diabetics', 'asthma' can be cured by using alternate medicines. I am not concluding nutritional balance is the only way. Perhaps, you may combine yoga + nutritional balance along with homeopathy or siddha to ensure good health. Bottom line is to STOP allopathic medicines that are very abusive by nature. This is my humble request to each of you to take care of yourself. You must stop habits that harm you, eat a light vegetarian food to lead a healthy life.

I would let you think about the life as it is an opportunity and wellness is your birthright. You can think about wellness now, and not after you're ill. It is essential for everyone to start from age of seven with simplified yoga exercises to streamline your body, mind. It will help you as an adult as it becomes a natural practice; instead of trying to force fit any sort of disciplines. You're born to live like a King and ensure you're able to reach the shores of your own kingdom; the heaven is inside you and waiting for your return back home. The magnanimous consciousness has manifested in you. It is imperative to keep body, mind healthy to reach the pinnacle of your own life. You're born with the unique opportunity to realize self and its lineage to nature. It will be a sheer waste of time indulging in mundane pleasures alone. Come on in and enjoy the ultimate freedom within deep yourself.

Blessed by the Divine!!!

Blessed by the Divine!!!
Blessed by the Divine!!!